Conflict in General Practice

This book is to be returned on or before
the last date stamped below.

Conflict in General Practice

Lynne A. Hobden-Clarke
Susan A. T. Law

FINANCIAL TIMES
Healthcare

FT HEALTHCARE
a Division of Pearson Professional Ltd
Maple House, 149 Tottenham Court Road,
London W1P 9LL, UK
Telephone: +44 (0)171 896 2424
Fax: +44 (0)171 896 2449
http://www.fthealthcare.com

First published 1997

A catalogue record for this book is available from
the British Library

ISBN 0-443-059365

Publisher: John Harper
Project Manager: Brenda Wren
Copy edited by: Samantha Evans, Sawbridgeworth
Indexed by: June Morrison, Helensburgh

Typeset by Saxon Graphics Ltd, Derby
Printed by Bell & Bain Ltd, Glasgow

Contents

The Authors

Lynne A. Hobden-Clarke

Lynne Hobden-Clarke started her career with Marks & Spencer plc, for whom she worked for fourteen years as a Personnel Manager. This gave her an insight into general business strategies, a keen understanding of profit and loss accounts, and financial targets and an enthusiasm for developing each individual to attain their full potential. In 1985 she moved into general practice as a Practice Manager in South Buckinghamshire, and in 1991 she also assumed the responsibility for the budget when the practice became first-wave fundholders. She had full responsibility for all aspects of organisation, personnel, finance, strategic planning and administration. During this time she was involved in a project to include practice managers in training practice assessment visits in the old Oxford Region.

In 1995 she moved to Norfolk and has been working as a freelance management consultant specialising in general practice. She acts as a trouble-shooter to practices who perceive that they have problems by undertaking organisational assessments, facilitating away days and advising on all aspects of management.

Lynne has lectured and written extensively on management issues and is an editorial adviser to a practice manager journal.

Susan A. T. Law MSc BA MRCGP

Susan Law was born in 1953 in Dundee where she was educated and went to University. Once qualified she tried her hand at hospital practice before seeing the light and completing her vocational training back in her native land. She then served as a medical officer in the Royal Air Force for fourteen years. During that time she became a widely experienced general practitioner and trainer. Latterly she was part of the Royal Air Force's Department of General Practice where she acted as Course Organiser and GP Tutor. After leaving the Royal Air Force in 1997 she plans a portfolio career combining medical teaching and medical practice.

Overview

WHAT IS CONFLICT?

Why is conflict so important that a book is written about it? Without it, our lives would be simple! However, conflict does exist and we all have to face and deal with it – it is part of our everyday lives. You could think of conflict as just like an illness which, if you understood it, you could manage, and that analogy may work. But it is important that we should not be introspective in looking for solutions to the problem of conflict, but should look outside the boundaries of our own professions in seeking answers to the problems that face us.

Conflict is defined in the Concise Oxford Dictionary as a fight or struggle, as a clashing of opposed principles and, also, as psychological distress due to the opposition of incompatible wishes. The word has been used to describe events as disparate as a world war involving millions of people and causing countless deaths, and a playground tussle between four-year-olds that ends in tears. It can describe the internal debate that takes place when we decide what we want to do. Conflict is a small word with great scope that can be used to cover a wide diversity of issues.

It is in a man's (and woman's) nature to fight to survive. The need for the species to survive has written this struggle into our very genes. In prehistory man hunted and the battle was against nature to win enough food to survive and to reproduce. Today we live in a 'civilised' society where struggles and conflict take place between fully trained and equipped armies, in childrens' playgrounds and across polished boardroom tables.

Conflict is part of our lives, it is an integral part of our interactions with other human beings. Used constructively it can generate good ideas and the impetus to succeed. Ignored or unrecognised it can cause psychological distress and destruction.

Conflict, in the sense of contrasting ideas, is not undesirable, because only through the expression of differences can good problem-solving take place. Teams that contrast, compare and discuss a problem often perform better than teams where there is little debate and the easiest answer is accepted to avoid conflict.

1. Introduction

Over recent years there has been an increasing awareness of conflict within practice teams, especially amongst the partners. A General Practitioner applying for a first partnership position can no longer assume that they will remain with that practice for their entire working life. Indeed, many would not want to do so. The dynamic nature of the National Health Service currently militates against longer-term planning.

We have seen some major external changes, for example the 1990 GP Contract and the introduction of the Purchaser/Provider split, which have exposed differences within otherwise settled partnership teams. These changes have been difficult to manage because they have centred around personal expectations, the way in which primary care is delivered and the traditional roles within the Health Service. The people most affected by some of these outside influences cannot be categorised by age, sex or background as the changes touch on personal agendas for a lot of these issues.

Many practice teams never discuss their motivation for being General Practitioners or the direction in which they wish the practice to progress, and such discussions are often only initiated as a result of the changes imposed from outside. Usually, these changes are threatening because they are implemented without anyone having the luxury of becoming part of the consultation process. For this reason, disharmony can surface in any practice at any time and involve any group of people.

AIMS OF THE BOOK

We aim to offer the reader one port of call to access information about conflict, however it manifests itself. Each chapter deals with a specific aspect and either the book can be read in its entirety, by those interested in the subject, or individual chapters can be used as reference tools in response to particular problems. We are aiming to offer not an academic masterpiece but a book written in unambiguous language which becomes a practical guide to managing conflict. There are many examples of real situations throughout the text as well as tables and charts to clarify issues.

Inevitably we do refer to other people's work when we feel it is particularly helpful and, on those occasions, full references will be given at the end of each chapter for those who wish to delve a little further.

The book is targeted to those working in general practice who have to manage conflict within their own environment. It will also be of interest to associated bodies like Health Authority staff and the NHS hierarchy, who could benefit from a greater insight into the peculiarities and idiosyncrasies of general practice, and will perhaps help them to understand why conflicts which they perceive as relatively simple can have such huge ripple effects.

Many practice managers are sympathetic but largely uninformed about the conflict that can occur between a doctor and a patient. We want to offer an insight into some of the mechanics of the consultation and help them to take a more proactive role in the delivery of care, and, at the same time, to become a more effective support for their General Practitioners. By the same token, many doctors simply cannot understand why a relatively routine personnel issue costs the manager so much time, effort and trouble to resolve. We hope that we can offer them an insight into the management of change on the more organisational issues that otherwise, perhaps, remain a closed book.

Another ambition is to provide practices, both managers and doctors, with an educational tool. This also has its place in the training of future GP Principals and future managers and perhaps in helping the newly appointed to integrate into a very complicated organisational structure. We hope that the readers will refer to the Chapter 11, where we give case studies and transcripts of consultations taken from real general practice. They offer a chance to actually explore the issues surrounding instances of conflict in a very safe and non-threatening way. They are designed to be used as training aids for the whole practice team, local practice-manager or action-learning groups, and GPs.

The final and perhaps the most important aim of the book is to actually bring conflict out into the open. We will be offering guidance on recognising danger signals in the behaviour of people working within general practice. Too often the first sign that there is a problem is when partners or practice personnel resign, leave or possibly try and split the partnership teams to gain what they want from their working lives. This book will be somewhere to go for advice on the issues that arise when a partnership fails and the practice manager is left with the dilemmas of how to cope with a new Partnership Agreement, how to resolve its legal status, how the staff are affected and how to manage a dysfunctional team.

When a major problem does emerge within a practice team, there is always the question, 'Could we have avoided this?' and the answer is often, 'Yes, of course we could.' We would like to remove the negative image that conflict has and show it as a very positive process because it is only from conflict that people start comparing their future needs and wants, and from this learn to manage change.

We would like to facilitate the transformation of practices from practices that have conflict into practices that use conflict to take themselves into the future, better prepared. Remember, from the grit comes the pearl!

WHY GENERAL PRACTICE IS UNIQUE

When considering their lot, GPs often compare themselves to other comparable professional partnerships within the commercial world. Here we outline some of the major differences, and explain quite clearly that this is akin to comparing apples to pears.

Professional partnerships

Let us take for our comparison a group of architects. The first and most striking difference is that the team tends to be of a single discipline. No permission is needed to set up a business and there are no government subsidies to offset any of the running costs. An architect is self-employed and available to any customer, and the fees for the work done are charged at the market rate or at whatever the market can bear. The range and the type of services that are delivered by that particular architect's practice is within the sole control of the principals as is their future development, financial security and longer-term aims and aspirations. Within most professional partnerships, the power base is actually much clearer than within a general practice partnership. The senior partner does not have that title through length of service, or any particular skills but because of his or her share of the business. The voting share is based upon the financial share and when one person leaves or, indeed, if they choose to sell part of their share, it can be bought by other people, thereby increasing their stake and their voting rights within their own organisation.

Even the appointment of a new partner is more flexible. It is commonplace to take on a prospective partner as an associate, or 'partner in waiting'. If a partnership vacancy arises there is full knowledge on both sides when an appointment is made. The existing partners have had the luxury of working with the candidates for a sufficient period of time to know their strengths and weaknesses and if the desired level of performance can be sustained. This facilitates better strategic planning and minimises the risk of offering a partnership position to someone who interviews well, but who turns out to be unsuitable when he or she joins the team.

There is no ceiling to the earnings in a professional partnership. There is a clear financial incentive for everyone to work hard to increase income and profit and to maintain a reputation for quality. Because customers are under no obligation to return to a specific architect, the practice must convince them that they deliver value for money.

NHS partnerships

The first major difference is that the team within the NHS tends to be multi-disciplinary. In fact, as we see more nurse practitioners and practice managers offered partnerships, this trend seems to be growing. A GP is self-employed. However, the main contract is with the NHS and a GP needs permission to accept NHS patients and approval before he or she can set up in practice. The reward for doing this is the receipt of a Basic Practice Allowance and other associated benefits. However, the income is then largely state controlled; indeed the 'claw back' system ensures that if more money is earned by GPs than was anticipated, then some of that is taken back in the following financial year. The current structure offers a 70 per cent reimbursement for approved staff, premises are provided via the cost or notional rent scheme and rates, such as Water Rates, are fully reimbursed. Computerised practices can receive a maximum of either 50 per cent or 75 per cent reimbursement if they choose to invest in a new computer system or to upgrade their old one.

The patients, or customers, are registered with an individual GP or practice, and their loyalty is usually high. It takes a great deal for the average patient to move to a different doctor. In reality, patients will often find excuses for the doctor who has not met their expectations, either in clinical or in organisational terms.

GPs are encouraged to be entrepreneurial and they can generate private income from other sources beyond their NHS Contract, for example, retainers and providing Personal Medical Attendant's reports and medicals to insurance companies. The nature of this state control of general practice makes GPs particularly vulnerable to the political climate, as the NHS tends to be a major vote winner, or vote loser whenever we have a General Election.

An NHS partnership is, in theory, truly democratic. In other words, every partner, irrespective of their contribution in terms of finance or time, has an equal voting share, which means that a newly appointed part-time principal has the same vote when it comes to a major issue as a very long-standing full-time partner. This obviously causes some resentment and it means that the power base is much more covert, and that the debating of major issues becomes more personal because people can only use their behaviour and personalities to gain perceived supremacy by gaining priority for their objectives before those of the other partners.

When it comes to taking on a new partner there are limited ways to guarantee success. In this situation, training practices have an advantage if they receive an application from a former GP registrar. They will either have personal knowledge of the candidate or be able to link in to the trainers' network to gain an insight and references. The other method of gaining prior knowledge is to employ locums or a doctor on the retainer scheme. Again, the practice can see for themselves issues like work rates, clinical effectiveness, administrative skills, team-working and special interests. Too often, practices advertise and interview unknown quantities and are vulnerable when making a final choice. A failure that results in a new partner resigning or being asked to leave is a difficult situation for all concerned.

Professional partnerships:

- single discipline, e.g. architects, accountants
- operates within a free commercial market
- no government subsidies to offset expenses
- voting by financial share
- clear hierarchy
- often an associate is 'promoted' to partner, with full knowledge on both sides.

General practice partnerships:

- income state-controlled
- reimbursement of some expenses
- vulnerable to government policies
- equal voting rights for all partners
- self-employed status, but contracted to the NHS
- some income from the private sector
- provide a service that is free at the point of contact

UNDERSTANDING PRACTICE TEAMS

There are very few medium-sized businesses in the UK, particularly in the commercial sector, where the company owners are also responsible for the income generation. Yet in general practice this is the accepted norm. The income of the practice comes almost exclusively from the doctor delivering a variety of patient services that are paid for by the Health Authority when the practice submits the necessary claim form or uses the GP/HA computer link. The average GP has also had to become an employer, potentially a property developer when it comes to extending surgery premises and a financier, especially if he or she are running a self-administered pension fund. There has been lots of scope in recent years for GPs to develop their entrepreneurial skills and some have even branched out into the teaching profession, voluntarily fulfilling the criteria to become a Training Practice and becoming actively concerned in the future development of the profession. All of these things rely upon each individual doctor's skills and interests and are not natural team activities.

Indeed, doctors spends many years learning to trust their own judgement, dealing on a one-to-one basis with each patient. Skills such as self-reliance and self-sufficiency in making a diagnosis and then following the treatment plan through are, quite rightly, highly regarded. The general practitioner may involve other health professionals in the community or refer the patient to a hospital consultant, but always retains responsibility for his or her patient. Yet, despite a training that emphasises the ability to work alone we expect a partner to walk out of the consulting room and instantly become a good team member. In other words, to change from sole responsibility to collective responsibility.

If you ask the average patient how they would describe a practice team, I am sure that many would resort to the TV stereotypes of Dr

Finlay's long-suffering receptionist and general factotum, Janet, who appears to have all the time in the world to talk to the doctor and to the patients, but nothing else appears to get done. The familiar sight of desks piled with claims forms and paperwork is conspicuous by its absence. The other popular stereotype is the District Nurse pedalling around the community on her old-fashioned bicycle complete with basket at the front. Of course, neither of these images could be further from today's truth. In order for doctors to fulfill their many obligations, they have found it essential to delegate the non-clinical tasks to other people.

When the New GP Contract was introduced in 1990, there was a dramatic increase in the number of practice nurses who were employed and who could take responsibility for the work involved in the health promotion clinics. This has also been true of the number of practice and business managers: the majority of GP partnerships, irrespective of size, now have a functioning practice manager. The value that these practices now place upon their manager has increased beyond all recognition. The first generation of practice managers, who were appointed in the late 1970s and early 1980s, were more usually the ex-senior-receptionist or practice secretary renamed. Things had moved on by the mid-1980s and skills from business that were once considered threatening and unnecessary actually became quite desirable attributes. The image of practice management has also changed dramatically in the last fifteen years and it is perceived as a very desirable career. A typical starting salary in 1997 would be, perhaps, in the region of £22,000–£25,000, rising to £30,000 and occasionally in excess of £30,000 where practices are very large or have a degree of difficulty, like a number of sites. Apart from being the highest-paid non-clinical member of the practice team, the manager has a very pivotal role in developing and enhancing the practice team. Some years ago, the team would have comprised GPs, perhaps a receptionist and secretary, a District Nurse and a Health Visitor (Fig 1.1). Today, the teams have become much bigger but also much more specialised and sophisticated (Fig 1.2).

The complexity of general practice and the 24-hour commitment has encouraged small or single-handed practices to group together to form larger partnerships, often working from purpose-built premises. This allows GPs to take advantage of economies of scale, especially when employing nursing and ancillary staff. In these larger practices the role and status of the manager is very clear.

In very large practices there may be additional layers of middle management, for example, office managers and deputy managers.

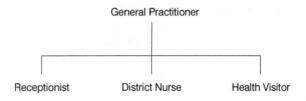

Fig 1.1 Traditional practice team – a typical 1970s structure

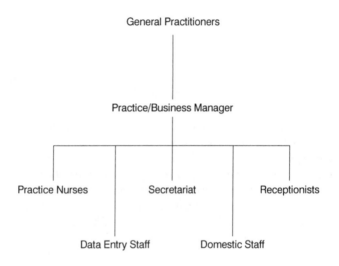

Fig 1.2 Practice team – a typical 1990s structure

Of course, in fundholding practices there is likely to be a fund manager and fundholding team. The relationship between fund and practice managers can be a potential source of conflict, especially if the reporting lines and responsibilities have not been made abundantly clear at the outset. This is explored more fully in Chapter 6.

Yet when we look at the wider team who deliver care and treatment to the patient we move into yet another level of complexity. It may be GP-led primary care, but the number of health professionals involved is almost endless.

Fig 1.3 gives an overview of the groups that a GP may liaise with in the course of a patient's treatment. This list is not exhaustive and will vary from practice to practice, especially if there are in-house facilities like a practice counsellor or alternative therapies. For those practices that are fundholding, this wider team will also

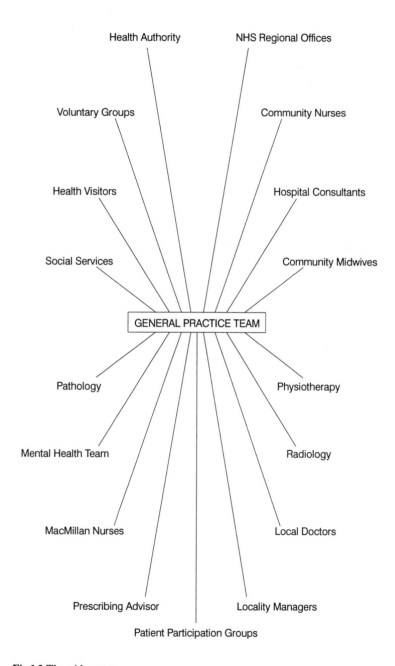

Fig 1.3 The wider team

include hospital business managers, contracting managers and the fundholding liaison personnel within the Health Authority and Regional Offices.

This large and sophisticated team brings with it a number of internal struggles because each individual within the team expects to feel valued and have the respect of his or her colleagues. There are a number of teams within teams, and the only method of judging the effectiveness of the wider team is the timeliness and quality of patient care. Too often, the complex structure of the teams, and politics can overshadow the purpose.

Building a strong practice team and maintaining it requires all the skills needed in a good personnel manager and will be covered in more detail in Chapter 4.

2. Symptoms of conflict

We are all familiar with the ways in which a doctor makes a diagnosis. It is a combination of everything the doctor sees, hears and perhaps instinctively knows from what is not said. It is exactly the same for the manager when diagnosing the health of his or her team. There may be a simple problem with one cause and one solution. Unfortunately these situations are quite rare and do tend to be the extreme cases. An example would be when a member of staff breaches a patient's confidentiality and is dismissed. More usually, the situations we find ourselves facing are more murky. There are, however, a number of behavioural indicators that will tell us when things are not going well and when the team is not working in harmony. The list is endless but given below are some of the more common types of behaviour that become apparent and demand our attention.

When we perceive one or a number of these behavioural indicators, it is essential to impose a sense of balance and objectivity before taking any action. There may be specific causes that will resolve themselves, and clashes of personality or an argument between team members often benefit from a night's sleep and time to allow the emotions to subside.

LACK OF INTEREST

This describes the attitude of the person who goes about his or her duties in a very dull and bored way. There is no hint of flair or even initiative to make the best of the job that he or she is doing and to take pride in it. It may be easily explained, for example if somebody is only three or four months away from retirement and they are simply biding their time to go on to do something that they are far more interested in. However, their withdrawal from the workplace in a mental sense may highlight a much bigger problem and a much bigger dissatisfaction.

Example:

Sheila is a receptionist who never smiles or joins in the routine banter in the reception area. She arrives exactly on time, and leaves exactly on time, she does her job adequately but without any enthusiasm. When asked to do anything extra she agrees, but her facial expression and attitude makes it clear that she is not pleased. When challenged she simply shrugs and says, 'If I must, I'll do it.'

UNEXPECTED BEHAVIOUR

Everyone establishes, what is, for them, their normal pattern of behaviour and this encompasses their attitude to work and to their colleagues. We can all think of people who are totally unbearable in the morning until they have had at least two cups of coffee and, conversely, those who are unfailingly cheerful, irrespective of the hour of the day or the pressures upon them. The warning signs are when people begin to behave out of character. This may describe the quiet person who never grumbles, who suddenly throws a tantrum, or it could describe the very loud, bubbly member of the team who suddenly goes very quiet and withdrawn. It may equally apply to the very obliging partner who takes every additional visit and emergency consultation with good grace, who suddenly digs in his or her heels and refuses to see another extra patient. (This is often combined with the doctor's retreat into his consultation room or a hasty exit out of the building.)

Example:

Alison has a wonderful temperament for dealing with the busy reception desk, telephone queries and difficult patients. She has endless patience and good humour and never gets annoyed, no matter how unrealistic the patient demands or expectations. One morning the other staff were amazed to hear her telling a patient on the telephone that his request was totally impossible and slamming the 'phone down.

LACK OF CO-OPERATION

There are many situations that can be overcome by goodwill, for example, a sudden shortage of staff or doctors due to legitimate illness or perhaps a family emergency. If the consequent additional workload is divided equitably between the remaining members of the team, then the situation becomes less fraught. The conflict in these situations arises when one or two members of the team are prepared to do more and others won't. The result is a huge inequality of workload with some members of the team feeling very put upon, and they are unlikely ever to be co-operative again.

Example:

Dr Graham is the newest of six partners, having recently completed his vocational training. He enjoys patient contact and is always willing to see 'extras' at the end of each surgery. After a few months he realises that the staff come to him first with any additional urgent consultation or visit, and he always takes it without complaint. His partners are therefore taking disproportionately less of this type of work. His innate sense of fair play tells him that this is wrong and he decides to be as reluctant as his colleagues to take extras. One day he sees that he is the only doctor doing home visits, the other partners having instructed the receptionists that they cannot do acute home visits for a variety of reasons. He decides to force the issue into the open and tells that staff that he cannot do any extra visits either, and leaves the building before anyone can tackle him.

EXCESSIVE DESTRUCTIVE CRITICISM

This does not include everyday grumbles about systems that fail us. Instead, it describes the behaviour of the member of the team who is unfailingly critical of everything without giving any new idea or initiative a chance. There are some people who can only make themselves feel better or perhaps give themselves more personal standing by trying to knock everybody else down. Unfortunately it can often extend beyond our performance at work and degenerate into a lot of personal criticism, perhaps typified by very unkind personal nicknames. It can be extremely wearing to work with somebody who persistently uses this approach. Sadly, a negative influence can be much more powerful than a positive one and a previously happy team can be completely overturned by one person who is consistently negative and critical.

Example:

Susan is an efficient fundholding data entry clerk and basically enjoys her work. In a previous job she was the manager of a small team and would really like to have this level of responsibility again. She feels that the practice manager is not firm enough, and criticises almost every decision made, claiming that anyone could do the job better. Instead of keeping her thoughts to herself she makes her feelings known to the other administrative and reception staff, and the practice manager's reputation is unfairly undermined.

LABOUR TURNOVER

There is always mixed emotion when somebody leaves an organisation. On the one hand we can rejoice in their reason for leaving and share their happiness if it is to await the arrival of a new baby or perhaps to move to a new area and a new life. The manager and partners may view the vacancy as an opportunity to change direction or bring new skills into the team, and be aware of the organisational benefits that labour turnover can bring. The sadness comes when we know that a familiar face is going to be leaving and a personality that we enjoyed working with is not going to be there any more.

If the person is leaving because they do not enjoy the job or because they are so unhappy that they feel they have no alternative, a completely different range of emotions comes into play. There may be feelings of guilt, that in hindsight the person was not given sufficient training or support to perform effectively. Their duties and responsibilities may have been changed quite fundamentally without them being part of the consultation process. People who resign under such circumstances have exercised their ultimate right to vote with their feet, and it is a public admission that a situation has become completely unacceptable. That is not to say that the organisation is always at fault, but rather that the process to resolve difficulties has broken down or was ineffective. The member of staff may have had totally unreasonable expectations and been unwilling to accept any compromise. It is possible that the whole team will become polarised between those for and those against what has happened and that there will be criticism of the management of the situation.

Example:

Ann joined the practice as a secretary having given assurances at her interview that she needed to work full-time for the foreseeable future. After three months she asked to reduce her hours, leaving every day at 2.30 pm. The practice manager explained that this was not acceptable because the doctors dealt with their paperwork between 3.00 pm and 4.00 pm, i.e. before afternoon surgery. As practice secretary she had to be available at those times, and the practice manager suggested a compromise of working until 4.00 pm each day. Ann said that this was impossible and resigned. Some staff felt that the manager should have agreed because Ann needed to be at home when her children came out of school, others felt that the practice was not a holiday camp and people had to be available when they were needed.

ABSENTEEISM

We all have occasions when we take time away from work because of illness. Most illnesses are entirely genuine and can be monitored by the standard employment procedures of self-certification, followed by a doctor's certificate if the illness persists for more than a week. The sort of absenteeism, however, that highlights a potential conflict is the sort that occurs frequently but is of short duration, i.e. odd days. Quite often there is a pattern that emerges over a period of time and it is important that everyone's absence record is monitored closely. The usual reasons given are the short, self-limiting type of problem like a headache, or a tummy upset. These are not serious enough to raise alarm and perhaps to get the manager out to go and visit the ill member of staff. A wall chart is an excellent way to plot any person's absence through illness. From this, it is instantly obvious if the pattern is, for example, every Friday or every Monday, or if a member of staff is always ill on a day that they usually have to do something they dislike. It also acts as an excellent deterrent if their ploy is likely to be noticed. This type of absence signifies that the staff member is unhappy enough to make the choice to stay at home rather than to face going into the practice, or that their working hours are unsuitable.

> **Example:**
> Sally hated working with Joan and they shared a shift on the reception desk every Thursday afternoon. Sally 'phoned in occasionally with a bad back. When the practice manager looked back at her absence record she was surprised to see that most absence occurred on Thursdays. When she placed a wall chart in the reception area and began to record everyone's absence Sally stopped 'phoning in with a bad back.

SARCASM

This a particularly difficult and manipulative symptom of conflict. It describes the behaviour of the person who hides behind a clever comment when in fact they have not got the courage to come out into the open and make a legitimate complaint or constructive criticism. By its sheer nature, it is very difficult to cope with as the protagonist so often wraps it up as humour, and the sarcastic person can keep the whole of the team on edge waiting for the next barbed comment and slowly undermine the confidence of any individual or of the whole group.

> **Example:**
>
> The practice manager asked the partners to be careful about their conversation in the reception area, because t' e staff were hearing snippets about confidential issues and these formed the basis of much speculation and scaremongering. One partner took exception to this and said loudly whenever he met another partner in reception, 'Be careful what you say, we don't want another telling off!' or, 'We can only talk about the weather in here.'

STEAMROLLERING

This describes the behaviour of the practice bully. This is the one who uses sheer force of personality or even their position within the practice to gain their own way. Reasoned argument is usually wasted because they simply refuse to listen, as it may result in them having to change their own approach. This unwillingness to be challenged can prevent the practice from progressing or taking on new initiatives, and although that may suit one individual it may hold back the rest of the team who think differently.

> **Example:**
>
> The senior partner was totally against computerisation of medical records and wished everyone to continue using a manual system. She had been a partner for 18 years and brought in a great deal of additional income from her occupational medicine activities. The other partners had all been in the partnership for less than five years and knew that the senior partner felt so strongly about maintaining manual records that she might leave. Whenever the topic was raised at practice meetings the senior partner would over-talk the others and produce spurious evidence that a manual system was best.

'THE GOOD OLD DAYS'

This attitude is typified by comments like, 'Well, it never used to be like that', and, 'But we have always done it this way'. It highlights the fact that someone is either threatened or challenged by the current state of affairs and by the likely future events. The piece of practice equipment that elicited most of these types of responses was the computer. The whole practice team was suddenly on a level playing field and everyone had to learn a new skill and cope with new technology. Some found this stimulating whilst others were probably terrified that they were going to be seen to be lacking.

INFLEXIBILITY

We can all think of people who stick rigidly to the demarcation lines of their job and, moreover, encourage everybody else to do the same. They tend to earn the unofficial title of 'the union shop steward'. What this type of behaviour really highlights is a complete lack of understanding of their role within the team and the fact that everybody's contribution has to be flexible for the whole thing to survive. There are those who arrive thirty seconds before they are due to start work and down tools at the exact minute that their shift ends, irrespective of what they leave half-done on their desk or the problems that they pass on to their colleagues. We rely heavily on flexibility and tend to train every member of staff in a variety of tasks, so one person who is unwilling to be flexible can cause disproportionate problems.

Example:

Jean is a district nurse and regularly visits an 80-year-old patient to dress her leg ulcer. The patient's 'over 75' check is due and the GP has asked Jean to undertake this on her next routine visit. Jean has been trained to do this and the locality manager is happy for her community staff to work closely with the practice nursing staff, sharing duties as appropriate. Jean refuses to do the elderly medical check, claiming that the doctor or practice nurse should do it and that she is too busy.

LOW MORALE

Morale is one of the attributes of a team that we judge in the negative. In other words, we tend to ignore it or take it for granted when it is there, but we always notice when it is missing. It can best be described as the complete absence of goodwill and an excess of criticism and grumbles. It is conveyed not just verbally but also by body language and facial expressions. One of the best tests of morale is in the organisation of a practice social event. If everyone refuses to go, there is obviously something very wrong. We spend so much time with our colleagues at work that the building of personal friendships is inevitable and it is sad if we have no desire to meet them away from the practice.

> **Example:**
>
> The practice manager was aware that the morale of the practice was at an all-time low. She decided that an 'away day' would be a good method of getting everyone away from the practice to discuss the problems and causes. When she proposed this at a practice meeting she received a very negative response from the partners, and this was echoed at a staff meeting when the part-time staff declared that they would not attend if it did not fit in with their normal working hours.

NON-ATTENDANCE AT MEETINGS

When a practice is facing a major decision, there are inevitably opposing views that need to be thrashed out before a consensus can be reached. The natural forum for these discussions is a practice meeting, but when the issues are becoming too painful, certain members can withdraw and refuse to attend the meetings. It may be simply because no vote can be taken in their absence or it may be that they cannot face any potential personal criticism of their particular viewpoint. It could, of course, be far more basic in that the meeting has been organised at a time when it is very unlikely that people can attend easily, and the manager has not been sensitive enough to reorganise the event. This could be combined with a sense of futility, in other words, a feeling that no matter how much discussion takes place, nothing ever happens.

> **Example:**
>
> Dr Allan had four partners: two were totally pro fundholding and two were anti. At the practice meeting a final decision was to be reached about entering a fundholding preparatory year. Dr Allan was quite open-minded about fundholding and could see the advantages and disadvantages quite clearly. He was asked to take an additional visit that he could do either before the practice meeting or afterwards. He did not really have enough time to go before the meeting, but did anyway. Thus he avoided having to make a decision, knowing that whatever opinion he adopted he would be ostracised by at least two of his colleagues.

PREOCCUPATION WITH TRIVIA

Some of the choices facing general practitioners are quite daunting, largely owing to their potential for failure. This is particularly true of concepts like fundholding or perhaps the appointment of a new partner. Fundholding can challenge the ideology of the practice and affect its whole ethos. Most GPs have been trained in the NHS, where all of the patient services are free at the point of delivery, and they cannot cope with the thought that they may have to ration care on financial grounds.

When it comes to appointing a new partner, the newcomer may well challenge a lot of the long-standing beliefs and traditions of the practice, which in turn can cause internal wrangling between the partners. Some people cope with this by avoiding the main issues and concentrating on the detail. For example, they expend a great deal of time and energy in examining one small part of the budget without looking at the bigger picture.

They may also fall victim to the 'halo effect'. This is when one really good part of a particular system or person overshadows any other weakness. The opposite of the 'halo' effect is the 'horns' effect. Just as we can allow ourselves to be deceived by an outstanding strength, we can be equally deceived by an obvious weakness. Colleagues are labelled because of an error of judgment on one single occasion and never allowed to live it down. The result is that any further contribution or suggestion is ignored, without being given any consideration at all. Too often decisions are made on this basis and insufficient time is given for proper research and validation before a decision is made.

Example:

One practice chose their computer system because it included colour screens, without considering any of its clinical functions or ease of use.

POOR PERFORMANCE

Just as in our personal behaviour, we also establish a norm in terms of our performance. None of us performs every part of our role equally and we all have strengths and weaknesses. However, an intervention is required when someone's standard of performance suddenly changes. It could be a very reliable person who suddenly starts making a lot of mistakes. This type of problem should be addressed informally in the first instance by the manager. There are a number of avenues to investigate. For example, there could be a problem with that person's domestic situation which means that they are preoccupied and their concentration has temporarily fallen off. It could also be, however, that another member of staff is not informing them and therefore they cannot do their work well, or there could be some sort of unresolved personality clash.

Example:

The book-keeper has always been meticulous in following up outstanding invoices and reconciling the bank statement at the end of each month. He works part-time having taken voluntary redundancy from a local bank. In fact, he was the practice's bank manager for some years. When he was on holiday the practice manager maintained the computer accounts and was surprised to find a desk drawer full of unentered information and cheques that had not been paid into the bank.

POOR PUNCTUALITY

No matter how good our intentions, everybody is late at some point in time. It may be for a perfectly valid reason, like the car breaking down – which is easily understood, easily explained and a one-off situation. In these instances, as the manager, we would expect a simple apology and for that person to offer to work on either in their lunch hour or at the end of the shift to make up for the time that has been lost. Poor punctuality becomes a symptom of conflict when it is regular and of a very small amount, or when no apology is offered and perhaps the member of staff tries to hide the fact that they have been late. This has to be tackled for a number of reasons. Firstly, no manager or partner can afford to be accused of favouritism in that they allow one person to conduct themselves in a manner that would not be tolerated from anyone else. Secondly, the group discipline has to be maintained. If one person's being late appears to be condoned, then there is every reason for the rest of the team to do exactly the same. Thirdly, the manager needs to be aware of any underlying problem that is preventing that person arriving on time. It may be short term and acceptable, for example, a sick child at home and having to make additional arrangements for child-minding, or it maybe a longer-term problem that requires some serious action about their employment.

The worst example of this would be a new member of staff who has accepted the job on a certain arrangement of hours that they know at the outset that they cannot fulfill. It could therefore be an attempt to alter their hours to suit them in the longer-term: this sometimes cannot be tolerated by the practice. No matter what the reason, the manager must be seen to follow up every incident of poor punctuality for the sake of the discipline of the team as a whole.

Example:

Carol was often late – but only when the manager was on holiday or attending a meeting. The other staff kept quiet for several months, taking the flimsy reasons that Carol gave for being late at face value. Eventually they got fed up with it and brought the situation to the attention of the manager. The manager appointed a deputy with specific responsibility to maintain staff discipline and report any instances of lateness to her. Carol stopped being late.

FORMATION OF CLIQUES

It is quite natural for like-minded people to want to join together. We see evidence of this in all sorts of clubs and societies. We are quite naturally drawn to people who share our outlook on life or with whom we have a common bond. This may take the form of family background, a similar domestic or financial situation or perhaps shared experience with a previous employer. This only becomes dangerous when it excludes the rest of the team. To be effective, a team needs to be able to take full advantage of differing views and opinions and the complete range of skills that is evident in each individual. To allow such polarisation to continued unchallenged will eventually undermine the effectiveness of the total unit.

Example:

Susan was a new receptionist and had settled in well. One day there was a general discussion about a difficult patient and she voiced a different opinion to the senior receptionist and one that was critical of the practice procedures. Susan found herself excluded from general discussions for some time and was made to feel foolish because 'she didn't understand the situation'.

BACKBITING

This is often the effect when cliques are allowed to form. In other words there are small groups of individuals who band together, who consider that their opinion on everything is the correct one and everybody else's opinion is wrong. If the practice regularly holds well conducted staff meetings where the person chairing ensures that every individual has an opportunity to state his or her point of view, then this situation is unlikely to continue for very long. However, in the absence of a proper forum, it is likely that these small groups of people will undermine one another by constant criticism.

> **Example:**
>
> Following on from the previous example with Susan ... The senior receptionist told all the other staff to be wary of Susan because she was a trouble-maker who criticised everyone else.

POWER STRUGGLES

It is naive to assume that the most senior or authoritative person within the organisation holds the most power. Anyone who has worked within a close-knit practice team will be well aware that the person who exerts most influence is not necessarily the manager or the senior partner. Power is a much more difficult quality to define and it can be used benignly or it can be used malignantly. An example of the benign style of power-brokering would be the receptionist who is very sensitive to all around her and alerts the manager and partners when another member of staff has a difficulty or perhaps a personal problem that she feels they could help with. An example of a malignant power-broker would be perhaps the receptionist who takes one comment about one person, repeats it to another and then stands back to watch the resulting chaos and bad feeling.

In Chapter 1 we discussed the idiosyncrasies of a partnership in general practice and the potential problems of this truly democratic organisation. The partners themselves are therefore not exempt from this particular type of power struggle, where they have only their force of personality and their behaviour to either persuade their colleagues that their point of view and their chosen course of action is going to be the correct one or coerce them into agreement.

> **Example:**
>
> Pippa babysits for several of the partners. It suits her because she has been widowed recently and finds her evenings lonely; she has worked for the practice for 20 years and enjoys her part-time work filing notes. The other staff are aware that Pippa babysits and that she tells the partners all the gossip. Therefore, if they want something done that they know the manager will disapprove of, they tell Pippa, knowing that she will pass it on when she next babysits. The partners raise the issue at the practice meetings and the practice manager is forced into the situation of seeming permanently negative because she argues against most of the proposals raised via this route.

NO ACCEPTANCE OF RESPONSIBILITY

Most people are very ready to accept responsibility for their actions when they have completed a task particularly well and the compliments are flying. The real test comes when things are going badly and a mistake has been made, and then we find that those people who were responsible suddenly fade into the background. The reasons for their reticence may be simple embarrassment or the fact that they are kicking themselves far harder than anybody else would do. A more disturbing reason for their behaviour would be that the atmosphere within the practice is such that they are to frightened to admit to a mistake. There maybe a history of public humiliation in the past when somebody else has tried something and failed.

Example:

Some medical records have been lost and they are needed urgently to provide a medical report to a solicitor. Eventually the notes are found, filed under the wrong name. Diane knows that she was the one who mis-filed them, but dare not admit to her mistake because the last time it happened the person was publicly chastised and asked to write out her alphabet and pin it on the wall by her desk.

REFUSAL TO CONFORM

Every organisation requires regulations and guidelines. The most simple example for every employee would be their job description, because from this come the parameters that give us our security and tell us when we are doing well and when we are not. For practice nurses there are clinical protocols that are agreed by the doctors to tell them what they should be doing for new patient checks and for chronic disease clinics. Whether we call this a job description or a clinical protocol, it is really a tool to allow people to use their initiative and to work to their full capability without wasting time checking with somebody else if they are taking the right course of action. Most people welcome these types of guidelines if they have been part of the consultation process and if they can see the validity of each new instruction. The conflict arises when these things are absent and people have a change imposed upon them that they do not understand or agree with, and therefore choose to ignore it. The partners of a practice are likely to be far more guilty of this type of behaviour than the general staff. This is partly because the decisions that they make impinge upon their own personal beliefs about the way they practise their medicine, and partly because they have an ability to work alone for a large percentage of their time. Therefore, the rest of the team will not know if they are not conforming to agreed practice policy.

The effect on the general staff when this happens is both confusing and time wasting. They may have any number of different systems in operation to do something as simple as booking home visits because each partner chooses to work in a completely different way to the rest. The margin for error increases dramatically and this was probably the reason for the practice trying to bring in a policy that everyone would adhere to in the first instance.

Example:

At a practice meeting the partners agreed that they would maintain the computerised summary on each patient's medical record. It was agreed that they could do the task more efficiently than anyone else as they read their mail in their consulting rooms and could enter the information daily. To avoid duplication, the notes summariser would stop updating the manual summary in the medical records. One partner disagreed with this decision, but agreed to go along with the majority view. She never entered any information into the computer summaries. When some of her patients left the area and their notes were recalled by the Health Authority it became apparent that the summaries had not been updated anywhere.

These symptoms of conflict are not exclusive to general practice. They are evident in any team of people working closely together where the team is not functioning well. Hopefully not many practices will suffer from all of the symptoms of conflict at the same time but it is likely that there may be one or two things working together that will alert the manager that they need to review the way that the team is managed. In Chapters 8 and 9, we shall be exploring some of the coping mechanisms and management techniques available to us so that we can channel this conflict and construct a much more productive working environment.

THE MANAGEMENT OF CHANGE

Most conflict within an organisation is a reaction to change. These changes can come from two directions. The first is an external force, and an example of this would the New GP Contract in 1990. This radically altered the way that GPs earned their income and brought in new concepts, such as target payments for certain services, which had been completely unknown to the medical profession before. Another example is a general election, when we face a possible change of government and then have to wait until the various changes they wish to make to the health service are introduced on the statute books. In both cases the changes are quite threatening because we are not part of the consultation and decision-making process and therefore feel very victimised as we are left to pick up the pieces. The second type of change is an internal force, and an example of this would be the need for a new partner or a new system to correct something that was going wrong. In these situations, the partners and the manager of the practice may make the decision and be fully involved in the total process, yet the staff, if care is not taken, may feel threatened by the outcomes of these decisions.

The way that we respond to these changes can vary enormously but basically we have two choices when it comes to management style (Box 2.1). The first is proactive: in other words, we look at the change ahead, prepare and plan for it. In this mode we actually retain control of the change. The second style is reactive, more commonly referred to as 'knee jerk' management. In this situation, we respond quickly to meet a deadline without giving the whole picture due consideration, and consequently we are in danger of making very poor decisions. This in turn creates more stress and we end up quite often going back and re-doing the whole thing properly. The price in terms of the team's health can be quite high. The decision-makers within the practice will be seen as ineffective and indecisive. The cost in financial terms can also be considerable when the amount of wasted training, new systems and even new equipment are brought into the equation.

Box 2.1   Management of change

Proactive – *anticipate, plan strategy, think consequences through logically, keep control of change.*
Reactive – *'crisis management', no plan for future impact or consequences, the change controls us as we look for an immediate response.*

No matter how we may prefer to work, we have to accept the reality of the NHS as a constantly changing environment, and we are vulnerable to changing legislation, increasing patient demands and the pressure that we put upon ourselves as we search for the highest standards of care that we can possibly deliver.

The first step in actually managing change is to think about it from more than one perspective. It may be patently obvious to us, as decision-makers, why we need an additional partner, a new member of staff or a new computer system. Yet to the other members of staff who have not been party to the decision-making process, these changes are far more likely to be seen as extra work and a threat to their own role and position within the organisation, and genuine fears may be aroused that the dynamics of the working environment that they enjoy will change. Box 2.2 'Differing Views of Change', will help a manager to think through the likely fears and questions that will be raised by the team.

Box 2.2   Differing views of change

Type of change	Management view	Employee view
NEW PARTNER OR MANAGER	Necessary to replace some-one who has resigned, died, was not suitable.	Will they make changes? Will they like me? Will I fulfill expectations?
NEW EQUIPMENT	Necessary to improve efficiency. Save staff time that can be redeployed.	Will I be able to cope? Will I be given sufficient training? Will I lose my job if it can be done better by machine?
NEW METHOD	Necessary to cope with imposed changes, meet targets or new initiatives.	Will my job be safe? Will I have to move offices? Will I become more or less valuable? Will my salary be affected?
NEW OBJECTIVES	Necessary to improve standards.	Are they trying to get more out of us? What happens if I can't cope? How reasonable are the new standards? Will my job satisfaction alter? Do I want pressure?
ADDITIONAL RESPONS-IBILITIES	Necessary to improve staff flexibility, achieve objectives and this means occasional reshuffles.	Will I be able to cope? Will the bosses still be pleased with my work? Will my colleagues be OK? Will I earn more money?

There is no substitute for accurate research when presenting the team with a potential change. This may take the form of background reading, checking on all the latest directives from the Regional Offices, or in-house audit. The essential point is that assumptions have to be double-checked with facts.

Too often in general practice we can make very major decisions on gut instincts. Whilst these can sometimes be correct, too often the margin for error is great. From this research we can actually begin to work out a number of viable options. Each option needs to be supported by a list of pros and cons and, wherever possible, a financial costing in the short term, medium term and the longer term. Some partnerships prefer to play the cards very close to their chest; in other words they do not communicate with the staff about what the likely outcomes are going to be until they are completely sure themselves. There are advantages and disadvantages in this method. The disadvantage is that the rest of the team rarely have the opportunity to become involved in the decision-making process and they are not given enough time to get used to the thought of a major change. The other reason for advising against this method is that the staff usually have the best ideas and most workable ones when it comes to making an alteration. The perceived advantage of the partners making the decision is that they are seen as giving clear direction and leadership.

However, there is a very fine line between this type of leadership and a dictatorial approach. The key to the whole process of managing change is to allow every single person to understand the reason behind it and then to involve those that are directly implicated in the change in the decision-making process; even those who are not directly involved need to have a level of information that allows them to move with the change rather than putting obstacles against it.

All of the above assumes that the doctors and the staff have an input into and an influence on the changes that are taking place within a practice, but there are times where this approach simply does not work. A good example would be an Health and Safety directive, where the practice manager must take a firm line to ensure that the practice operates within the given legislation. The consequences of not doing so could be a prosecution.

Example:
Imagine the situation if the fire alarm goes off and we start to negotiate with patients and staff to leave the building when their lives may be in danger!

In conclusion, we must consider each change carefully and allow enough time to discuss the likely impact and agree the best course of action. On some occasions it will be appropriate to consult the whole team, on others we will be required to take a firm line and issue a directive.

FURTHER READING

Hasler J C et al 1991 Handbook of Practice Management. Longman Group
Pringle M et al 1991 Managing Change in Primary Care. Radcliffe Medical Press

3. Conflict with patients

We rarely see patients when they are well and happy. Even if they are attending for a routine health promotion check there is likely to be an underlying tension or unspoken fear about the discovery of an undetected illness. Consequently, any patient that comes into professional contact with a member of the practice team is often ill, worried or feeling threatened. Those with a mental illness may be confused or unpredictable. We are accustomed to helping the newly bereaved cope with their loss and the inevitable paperwork and legal procedures. All practices have a minority of patients undergoing treatment for drug and alcohol abuse, and these may arrive at the surgery drunk or under the influence of an illegal substance. In short, we have to be ready for anything. General practice is led by patient demand. It is not like a manufacturing production line where resources can be matched exactly to output. We plan to a norm, which means extreme pressure on resources when patient demands are higher than average and spare capacity when demand is low. This implies that our staff, personal attitudes and practice systems need to be equally responsive and flexible. In this chapter we will follow the progress of a patient from their arrival at the surgery premises to the conclusion of the consultation. We will highlight potential pitfalls and ways in which we can reduce the potential for conflict with the patient.

THE RECEPTION AREA

The reception area is the shop window of the practice. The initial impression we make on patients and visitors will have the greatest and longest-lasting impact. A cluttered and disorganised reception desk will signal inefficiency to the patient, irrespective of the quality of clinical care.

It is a good idea to walk around the practice premises occasionally and view the surroundings objectively, making clear assessments of the endearing or discouraging points seen from a patient's perspective.

We can reduce the potential for conflict with patients if the atmosphere is welcoming and calming. This will be more difficult in premises where space is at a premium, but the same principles apply. In some geographical areas, e.g. inner cities, security of staff from violence is a priority and this will be dealt with later in this chapter, but again, a balance should be possible.

When asked what an ideal reception area requires to radiate an aura of welcome and calm, we would probably bring expensive hotel lobbies to mind, or even private hospitals. Few practices have the funds or space for such ambitions. We have more practical considerations, like vomiting children and the incontinent. Comfortable fabric-covered sofas may be pleasing to the eye but vinyl is more durable and easier to clean!

It is within the scope of every practice to have clean, pastel-coloured walls and to maximise the amount of natural daylight with pale, vertical or horizontal blinds. Murky corners can be brightened with spotlights.

Seating that is padded helps the patients to remain comfortable, especially if they have a long wait. Fixed seating will keep the waiting area tidier than individual chairs, which get moved around. The arrangement of seating can also make a difference. One large room with chairs around the edge so that everyone can see everyone else can be embarrassing, especially for the distressed patient. A formation which divides the waiting room up can provide a more informal atmosphere and offer protection for those seeking anonymity (Fig 3.1). Strategically placed plants can soften a stark area, and larger ones make excellent room dividers and screens.

If patients are kept waiting for longer than they consider reasonable to see a doctor they become irritable. The waiting area should, therefore, offer some distractions. The notice boards are an excellent way to convey health-related information in a way that is pleasing to the eye. Too often posters and notices are pinned on top of one another, out-of-date material is left on display and the overall effect is chaotic. To delegate one person to be responsible for the notice boards is one solution. Their brief should be clear and if they can dedicate each board to a theme that changes two or three times a year, the regular attendees will gain new information.

Example of an impersonal waiting room:

Entrance to/from the reception desk and consulting rooms

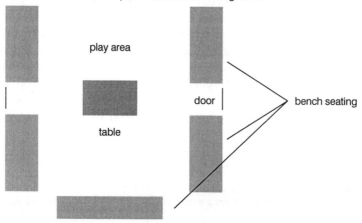

Example of a well planned waiting room:

Entrance to/from reception desk and consulting rooms

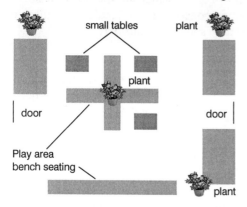

Fig 3.1   Waiting rooms

The traditional distraction in a waiting room is reading materials. Most magazines are donated by patients when they have finished with them, hence a predominance of stuff that is several months old. The range can also be limited or biased towards women's interest and few general topics that appeal to both sexes. It may be an idea to order a couple of daily newspapers for the waiting room, ensuring up-to-date reading matter. Most busy people would welcome a chance to sit down and read a paper in peace.

The measures a practice takes to create a pleasant and relaxing area for patients before they consult a doctor or nurse can be completely destroyed by boisterous or unhappy children. The former may run amok and the latter cry constantly. Attention must be paid to the needs of our younger customers by the provision of a play area and toys. Bearing in mind the amount of use and abuse that toys will receive, they should be robust and clean, with regular checks to throw out broken or potentially dangerous ones. Play areas should be situated in a quiet corner away from the main seating to minimise the disturbance to other patients.

> One of the most effective play areas is a miniature table and chairs with activity toys and children's books, plus a sign asking children to put away the toys when they have finished with them. The children may not be able to read, but it proves a useful reminder to accompanying adults

The use of pre-recorded video tapes is becoming more popular. They can play health related topics or a programme of cartoons to amuse children. Some companies offer a payment to practices who agree to show tapes on health topics which are sponsored by advertising. These have mixed responses, but the medium of videos to create the desired atmosphere should be considered.

Scenario:

Mrs Smith has booked an appointment for her four-month-old baby who has cried constantly for three days. She also has a three-year-old toddler who has to go with her because she cannot find a suitable person to baby-sit for an hour.

Experience 1:

Mrs Smith could not see a secure area outside the main entrance to leave the pushchair. She had difficulty getting through the swing doors with a pushchair, baby and toddler. She checked in and sat down on a hard plastic chair. All the other patients were sitting around the edge of the room staring at a table in the middle piled high with dog-eared magazines. The toddler was bored and started running around and shouting. She tried to calm him down, but failed. The baby cried continually and she could see the disapproving looks from the other patients. Mrs Smith already felt tired, worried about her baby and embarrassed at her toddler's behaviour and her inability to distract him. When the receptionist apologised that the doctor was running thirty minutes late, Mrs Smith lost her temper, shouted at the receptionist and stormed out.

Experience 2:

Mrs Smith left the pushchair in a designated pram park and walked through the automatic doors into reception. She checked in and chose to sit near the children's play area. Her toddler made straight for the toys and played contentedly. The baby cried continually and she was grateful to find a seat that offered some seclusion from the other patients. When the receptionist apologised that the doctor was running thirty minutes late, Mrs Smith was not pleased but she continued to wait.

An additional tension can be created by the method used by doctors and nurses to summon patients into their consulting room. There is no doubt that a doctor or nurse going to the waiting area to meet a patient starts the consultation on a positive note. The patient is more likely to relax in the knowledge that they will not be overlooked. Contrast this with an intercom or remote method of calling a patient. Those in the waiting room have to be alert and watchful, knowing that if they miss their turn they will face a longer wait. Instead of defusing tension, it may increase it.

THE IMPORTANCE OF TRAINED RECEPTION TEAMS

We are all familiar with the description of 'dragon' for a doctor's receptionist. Yet to combat this type of reputation we must understand the receptionist's role. He or she is piggy in the middle. If the doctors feel overburdened they blame the receptionists for booking inappropriate appointments, if the patients cannot see the doctor within what they consider a reasonable time they blame the receptionist for not fitting them in.

The receptionist's responsibility is to administer the practice systems effectively, and he or she should not be blamed when the policy decisions are ill-advised. We shall examine such conflicts with staff in some detail in the next chapter.

Telephone access

The first hurdle for the patient wishing to make an appointment with a doctor or nurse is usually telephone contact. We are in an age of technology that can transform communication, yet many practices still only have one line to book appointments. It may be a conscious ploy to suppress patient demand, and hence workload, but it is far more likely that no one has audited the patients' views or difficulties.

A simple survey form left in the waiting room for patients to complete is both cheap and effective (Box 3.1). Some practices may be aware that patients find telephone access difficult and annoying but choose to ignore it because of the financial implications of purchasing a new telephone system.

Box 3.1   Telephone Questionnaire

How many times did you ring the practice
before you got through?   _____ times

Were you put through to the correct department or person
(tick one answer only)
a) within one minute   _____
b) within two minutes?   _____
c) longer than two minutes?   _____

Did the person answering the telephone understand
your query?   YES/NO

Did you have to be transferred to another person to answer
your query?   YES/NO

How would you rate the telephone access to the practice?
(tick one only)
a) easy, can always get through   _____
b) usually easy, sometimes have to try more than once   _____
c) difficult, often have to try several times   _____

General comments:

When patients gets through on the telephone what sort of impression is made? Are they greeted with a cheerful voice? Are they asked to telephone a different number because they are trying to make an appointment on the enquiry line? Do they have to repeat their problem to several people until they speak to the right one? Are they left hanging on with no explanation or apology? Does the telephone ring and ring before it is answered? Is the patient offered guidance on the best time to telephone for a specific query, e.g. between 2 pm and 4 pm for test results?

The average patient may take these things in their stride, but some will become annoyed and vent their frustrations on the person answering the telephone.

Not many people favour the 'Hello, this is Julie on reception at the Woodlands Health Centre, how can I help you?' type of response when answering the telephone. It not only increases the amount of time spent dealing with each call, but may also confuse the patient enough to make them forget what they wanted for a few seconds. A more simple 'Good morning, Woodlands Health Centre', is enough to convey a helpful attitude and reassure the patient that they have dialled the correct number. Should the call be an emergency, then precious seconds have been saved.

The biggest frustration when telephoning any organisation is gaining speedy access to the correct person to deal with the query. We all know how annoying it is to explain our problem, only to be told that we were speaking to the wrong person and need to be transferred. We get put on hold for varying amounts of time and explain our problem all over again. The whole process may be repeated, by which time we feel thoroughly hostile and convinced that no one knows what they are doing or cares.

There are a number of ways to deal with calls on hold. Often taped music is played but there is no substitute for an human voice cutting in at regular intervals to explain the situation and offering options, e.g., 'The practice manager's line is still engaged, would you like to continue holding?'

To really help the incoming caller the receptionists need to be fully informed about everyone's responsibilities within the practice and their daily schedule. It sounds far more efficient to say, 'The practice manager is in a meeting, but should be free at 2.30 pm'. Taking a message is always an option and can improve efficiency if done well. However, if the practice has a reputation for inefficiency, the patients may be reluctant to do so. It is worthwhile investing appropriate resources to deal with telephone contacts and structuring the staff rota in such a way as to have someone available to deal with the complicated and time-consuming queries. Most switchboards are so busy that the person answering the telephone is unlikely to have the time. A pad beside the telephone specifically for messages is a good idea to instil a measure of discipline and standardisation.

Box 3.2   Telephone messages

```
Date: ..................................................
Time: ..................................................
Message for: ........................................
From: ...................................................
Message:


Contact telephone no: ........................
```

The type of message format in Box 3.2 can be used for everything including requests for home visits. Alternatives are messages jotted on Post-it notes and scraps of paper, not recommended because they are easily lost. Certain messages from patients are extremely important and their mismanagement may result in a doctor being accused of being in breach of their Terms of Service, e.g. a visit request getting lost. It is becoming more popular for doctors to offer telephone consultations or contact patients requesting a home visit to verify both problem and need. This requires that all staff know when doctors will be available for such calls and for the doctors to be free at the agreed time.

General practice has to be cost-conscious and encourage patients to make the telephone calls. This system works well if patients are given clear guidance about when to 'phone and the name of the person they need to speak to; it works badly if a busy receptionist just tells them to call again later and the patient makes several calls before they can get the information they need.

Scenario:

Mrs Black has had a blood test and wants the result.

Experience 1:

Mrs Black telephones the surgery the day after the blood test was taken, at 9.00 am, to be told the test result is not available. She telephones every morning and on the third day the receptionist tells her off for 'phoning at the busiest time and says to ring back in the afternoons. Two days and telephone calls later, she is told her result is fine and nothing needs to be done.

Experience 2:

When the nurse takes the blood test she explains that it will take a week for the result to come through. Also that, as the results arrive at lunch time, it is best to 'phone after 2.30 pm.
Mrs Black makes one telephone call the following week and is told her result is fine and nothing needs to be done.

Arrival at the reception desk

The first impression of the reception desk is purely visual. A clear desk with a plant or vase of flowers conveys calm efficiency. A cluttered desk with an array of charity collection boxes, patient leaflets and muddled posters and notices conveys disorganisation. Neither impression is necessarily an accurate portrayal of the practice but they are part of the opinion-forming process of the consumer. The positive image can be enhanced by staff uniforms or an obvious dress code.

Sadly, protection of staff has become essential in certain geographical areas and grills or glass barriers may confront the patient. These do little to reduce the potential for conflict, but are a part of everyday life and the physical safety of staff must take precedence over aesthetics.

The second impression is the attitude of the receptionist, which can either calm or antagonise. Patients will usually respond with the same tone and demeanour as the receptionist. The team must be trained in public relations and their part in enhancing the reputation of the practice stressed. There are many excuses for a grumpy or abrupt receptionist, e.g. illness or domestic worries, but none are acceptable, even if the alternative is moving staff temporarily to other duties. Their main purpose is to be helpful, kind and calm. An anxious patient will be reassured by this approach, not annoyed or made to go through unnecessary bureaucratic hoops.

Certain groups, like the elderly or hard of hearing, need lots of patience and someone who can provide clear explanations without being patronising.

To be well trained, the receptionists need clear guidance to follow. There should be a manual at hand to remind staff how to deal with each request, from booking a nurse appointment to taking a private medical insurance claim form. So much conflict can be avoided if receptionists make realistic promises about the amount of time that it will take to perform certain tasks or clearly explain fees that are chargeable for non-GMS work. They also need the support and back-up of the partners and manager. If they are following a policy agreed by the partnership and a patient takes exception and complains, it is the policy that needs to be reviewed and criticised – not the member of staff. By the same token, if a doctor takes exception then the same applies. Too often the reception team bear the brunt of everyone else's disgruntlement.

Occasionally, patients arrive in a very distressed state. The sensitive receptionist will offer them somewhere to wait away from the general area, usually an empty consulting room or office. This contains the situation and prevents distress from escalating into embarrassment or anger.

Scenario:

Mr and Mrs White have been married for over fifty years and they are both in their seventies. Mr White had been ill for some time and died quite unexpectedly. Mrs White and her son have come to the surgery to collect the death certificate.

Experience 1:

Mrs White goes to the desk and the receptionist asks how is her husband? Mrs White bursts into tears and her son gets angry that the receptionist does not know that his father has died and they want the death certificate. Mrs White and her son are left standing at the desk while the receptionist looks for the certificate. It cannot be found and the doctor concerned is away until the afternoon. The receptionist tells Mrs White that there is nothing she can do and to come back later. They return later, the doctor has not arrived and the certificate is not available. Mrs White's son loses his temper and demands to see the manager. At this point the GP arrives and says the certificate was on top of his desk as he knew Mrs White would be calling for it.

Experience 2:

The GP leaves a note on reception to inform the staff that Mr White has died and the death certificate is on his desk. When the receptionist sees Mrs White and her son, she offers her condolences and shows them into an empty consulting room while she fetches the certificate. She also checks that Mrs White knows where to register her husband's death and the times that the Registrar will be available. Mrs White and her son ask the receptionist to convey their thanks to the staff.

Keeping all staff informed is a vital part of the process to avoid conflict with patients. The reception team needs to be trained in all routine systems and procedures, and especially in sensitive duties, like the scenario described above.

CONFLICT WITHIN THE CONSULTATION

A consultation with a doctor is an event in most patient's lives. A doctor may see 200 patients a week, but a patient consults on average only two or three times each year. Each party gives the events a different significance. For the consultation to be a success, both participants must communicate and, at the very least, negotiate a satisfactory outcome to the occasion. Unfortunately, many consultations involve conflict between the patient and the doctor. Many things can cause conflict to arise, an angry patient, an unhappy doctor or just a simple misunderstanding. This section will look at some of the areas that can cause conflict and will offer some suggestions for avoiding or managing them.

Communication failure

What is communication failure? It happens to us in all sorts of situations. The causes can be obvious or complex but it exists when to a greater or lesser degree a consultation ends unsatisfactorily.

Language

An obvious cause of communication failure is differing spoken languages between the patient and the doctor. The resulting misunderstandings could lead to frustration and anger in both patient and doctor. This is perhaps obvious when dealing with a multi-ethnic group or with doctors whose primary language is not that of their patients, but even when dealing with people whose mother tongue is English problems can arise. Dialect can be a real problem; in moving south or north the accent changes dramatically and it is easy to miss the nuances that patients try to get across. English usage varies not only

> I remember moving to Sheffield from rural Scotland: what did 'mardy' mean? It means the same as 'girney' in Dundee and 'hingy' in Newcastle – a general unwellness with no specific illness.

across the counties but within social class; some swear words are used as general purpose adjectives rather than with intent to offend, others are used for dramatic effect. Conversational style must also be remembered: patients who are reticent, rambling or vague can be extremely irritating to the doctor just as vague and woolly doctors irritate their patients.

Just as dialect or usage can be a barrier to communication and a cause of conflict so can jargon. As a profession, doctors use lots of jargon, often unintentionally and with no wish to confuse their patients. Using jargon does not matter when both parties know the meaning of the words but in the doctor–patient relationship it is usually the patient who ends up frustrated

> What is a heart murmur? To a doctor it is a noise produced by turbulent blood flow that may or may not have any significance. When doing routine medicals I have often found a murmur that has proven to be insignificant; however, using the term 'murmur' has serious connotations to the average patient and I now try to use the expression 'unusual noise' which has fewer worrying connotations.

by their inability to get the doctor to explain things in clear and simple English. This means that jargon must be used carefully within the consultation. Doctors should be conscious of the potential difficulties of jargon and must be sure at the end of every consultation that any jargon used has been carefully explained. Failure to do so could lead to misunderstanding and conflict.

There is no easy solution to the problem of language, but it is important to be aware of the issues that misunderstanding or failure of communication can cause. Doctors should be conscious of the issues of dialect, usage and jargon and should become familiar with local colloquialisms and idiosyncrasies.

Relationship

Communication failure can also arise when a relationship is not established early on in the consultation. It takes both parties to establish a good doctor–patient relationship but when the patient arrives it is incumbent upon the doctor to provide a pleasant and welcoming environment.

The formation of that relationship begins when the patient tries to make an appointment. The helpfulness or otherwise of the staff who answer the telephone and the length of time before the appointment both influence the formation of the relationship. Unnecessary inquisitiveness on the part of a receptionist and a three-week wait for a routine appointment are not conducive to strong relationships. The ambience of the reception area and the manner of the reception staff add other bricks to the foundations. An unkempt waiting room with wooden benches or offhand staff may adversely effect the relationship that is forming.

Then the doctor enters the equation; poor time-keeping can cause frustration and anger, particularly if the patient has had to make a special effort to see the doctor. Although aware that doctors can run late, when lateness is excessive or becomes a regular event some patients do take it as a personal insult. This can often be defused by arranging for the staff to provide information about any delays, or by a simple apology from the staff or the doctor. If the doctor fails to greet the patient pleasantly or uses inappropriate body

When I am running late, each time I go to the waiting room to collect a patient I offer a general apology to all those waiting and let them know that I am running late. If patients are sent through to the doctor by the receptionist this could equally well be reception's responsibility.

language a barrier can be raised which can block communication. Even the layout of the office can make or mar a consultation. In a surgery where consulting takes place across a vast expanse of desk, communication becomes one-sided, from doctor to patient, and the patient's resulting frustration may lead to conflict.

Appropriate body language is an additional precursor to a successful relationship. Our bodies tend to reflect our inner feelings. When we are confident and comfortable we tend to sit in a relaxed posture, our arms are unfolded and rest relaxed in our laps. We are receptive to what the patient brings. However, a closed posture, with arms folded, a hunched back, failure to make eye contact, more attention paid to the computer than to the patient equate to, in the patient's eyes at least, lack of interest! An open posture, eye contact, attention and as Carl Rogers says 'unconditional positive regard' are all factors that help form a strong working relationship.

Carl Rogers used the expression when he discussed mentoring and adult learning, but 'unconditional positive regard' applies equally to the doctor–patient relationship. The words may sound like jargon, but if you think about their meaning they become easy to understand. 'Unconditional' means you put no conditions on your regard: if the patient is smelly, rude or you just dislike him or her you must try not to allow these factors to influence your work. 'Positive regard' encompasses a positive outlook towards your patient, disregarding the negatives as far as possible, which if practised will allow you to overcome your own failings and to look at the situation without the clouds of stereotyping or bias to affect your practice. Care should be offered and administered with the same respect, dignity and kindness for every patient seen.

Additionally, it is important that the correct balance is struck within the doctor–patient relationship. Traditionally doctors have been seen as the father figure and have often assumed a parental role within the consultation. This may work if the patient is comfortable with and assumes a childlike role. Unfortunately if the patient wishes to be treated in an adult fashion and to have a relationship of equals with his medical adviser, his consultation with a paternal doctor will only end in disaster. Medical training is now trying to encourage doctors to become partners with their patients during the consultation process so that the dynamics are that of adult expert (patient about himself) and adult expert (medical practitioner) reaching a satisfactory solution to a consultation. These theories are further amplified in Berne's *Games People Play* and Tuckett's *Meetings between Experts*.

Culture

While language difficulties are the obvious result of a meeting of two different cultures, there are many other issues that can impede communication. Different ethnic groups have different health beliefs, which may conflict with western medicine as we understand it. This is particularly the case with psychiatric illness in cultures where a belief in spirits or possession is extant. Western medicine would classify the Caribbean conditions of the 'evil eye' and 'voodoo death' as phobic states, while in Malaysia spirit possession and 'amok' refer to conditions we would describe as dissociative states. Some Asian groups associate depression with possession by an evil spirit and use violence as a way of exorcising that spirit.

Different cultures react differently to their health experiences. A classic study in the USA, quoted by Cecil Helman in *Culture, Belief and Illness*, compared the perceptions of pain felt by three cultural groups. The Italian Americans tended to exaggerate their experience of pain and to emphasise the immediacy of the pain. The Jewish Americans also exaggerated their experience of pain but were much more concerned with the meaning of that pain. The third group, the Protestant 'old' Americans reacted by withdrawal from the pain and assumed a 'detached' air, a stiff upper lip attitude.

Although western medicine has moved away from the belief that health is related to temperature balance, some Chinese and Asian medical practices still hold to these beliefs. Foods and medicines have the symbolic power of hot and cold and are consumed appropriately to balance the temperature. This can cause severe vitamin deficiencies in post-partum women whose diet may be unbalanced because of this belief.

While the differences described in these examples do not themselves cause conflict, it is important for us as professionals, to understand how easily a misunderstanding can arise if the doctor and the patient are of two different cultures. If the explanation of a disease or a treatment is not understandable within the context of the patient's belief system it is likely that misunderstanding, confusion, non-compliance and conflict will arise.

Both the doctor and the patient belong to a 'culture', and while we have talked of the patient's culture it is important not to forget the doctor's cultural experiences. A doctor trained in parts of Europe will automatically prescribe headache remedies to be taken by suppository. This is not common British practice and the average British patient will be expecting some tablets. This mismatch of

I am reminded of an Asian trainee who worked with my mother. He acknowledged how difficult it was for him to say, 'I don't know'. His culture expected the expert to behave as such and to admit lack of knowledge was to admit failure, which resulted in loss of face. At home such behaviour would cause his patients to seek other experts and he would soon have no patients to see.

expectation is likely to cause non-compliance: a source of irritation to the doctor and frustration to the patient, who has not had his or her problem solved. Again, there are no easy solutions to the issues that differing cultures raise. It is incumbent upon us as professionals to be aware of the issues and to recognise potentially threatening situations, if and when they arise.

Stereotyping

Stereotyping is not perhaps often considered in the doctor's day-to-day existence but we all use stereotyping as a short cut. We make assumptions from minimal information and then assume that these assumptions will hold good across a population. The classic medical stereotype is the holder of 'thick notes'. Individuals with thick notes are usually assumed to be female, have multiple unsolvable psychological problems, are often overweight and generally cause a 'heartsink' feeling in the doctor. The patient must nevertheless be seen, and the construction of the overwhelmingly negative stereotype that goes with thick notes is not a good foundation upon which to build a productive relationship. We don't just stereotype holders of thick notes: we stereotype the elderly, the overweight, the patient who has had a psychiatric problem, the homosexual and the patient with HIV infection. We may not categorise people intentionally, but it is a mechanism that our brains use to make judgements often from very little information. While it can be a useful tool it can also be very dangerous. Stereotyping an anxious middle-aged woman with a past history of a depressive illness may lead you to suppose that she comes to see you with a recurrence of her psychiatric problem or for

A colleague told me of a case of a frequent attender, a fat middle-aged woman, with thick notes and a history of depression. For years she had been coming in complaining of headaches, tiredness and lassitude for which no reason had been found and which had been diagnosed as probably psychiatric in origin. It was when a new, unbiased partner arrived who listened to her and who examined her thoroughly that the signs of hypothyroidism emerged. On treatment she is a changed person.

reassurance. It may cause you to miss the importance of a new problem and even to misdiagnose a potentially serious illness.

Unrealistic expectations

Amongst the most difficult causes of conflict to resolve is unrealistic expectations on the part of the patient and sometimes even the doctor.

Unrealistic expectations can be as simple as expecting a prescription of antibiotics for a sore throat. Many GPs still prescribe antibiotics for sore throats: there is little evidence to suggest they are of much value but similarly there is little evidence to suggest that taking an additional course of antibiotics will actually harm an individual. Today's thinking inclines to giving advice for sore throats and only prescribes antibiotics if a sore throat lasts more than a few days or is associated with other signs of illness. Given that, what does the average doctor do when faced with a patient with a mild sore throat and little else in the way of symptoms? Often the patient has been seen before with similar sore throats and has had antibiotics on those occasions; the patient probably expects antibiotics again. To prescribe or not to prescribe?

Failure to prescribe could involve the doctor in a conflict situation, particularly if the patient feels that the antibiotics will work and that they are being denied their dues. Health education in a 10-minute appointment slot is not always possible, although in this case some time spent explaining the pros and cons of treatment may save additional time at a later date.

A common expectation that is often a source of conflict is referral to the hospital. Many patients are not aware of the battery of investigations that the average GP has at their finger tips. They tend to expect referral to specialists particularly if a problem has not resolved in the time scale they expect. Time is a great healer and it is surprising how often problems resolve while patients are on the waiting lists for their local hospital. Another issue is the time spent on a waiting list. This can be quite considerable for some specialties. Patients tend to assume that a referral will get a fairly prompt response. An instant response is a cause for

I remember a patient coming to see me, he had a history of severe indigestion and his expectation of the consultation was a referral to hospital. It took some time to explain to him that the tests he needed could all be organised from the surgery much more quickly than if he was referred to a consultant.

concern: something dreadful is wrong; as is a date for the middle of next year: how am I going to cope for the next nine months? These potential sources of conflict should be explored within the consultation and the way forward should be negotiated jointly.

Unrealistic expectations on the part of the doctor may be a more difficult problem. An example is the obese patient who cannot lose weight even though she 'starves' herself. The doctor is unrealistic if he expects ever to help this woman become thin, and banging his head against a brick wall will only lead to frustration and conflict. Very often, the best that can be offered is a contract within which a limited degree of weight loss has been negotiated and which can be monitored. If appropriate, praise can be given by the doctor. There is no point in the doctor spending vast amounts of time chastising this woman; she knows she is overweight but no amount of chastisement is going to change the situation. It will only lead to a poor relationship and conflict with her doctor.

The patient on benzodiazepines who is reluctant to give up her tablets may also cause unrealistic expectations. Patients who have become very reliant upon their drugs may find it very difficult to give up. If the doctor rushes in and demands that the patient stop taking their medication forthwith he or she is doomed to failure. Again a contract which is feasible and acceptable to both parties has to be negotiated. Coming into conflict over the issue is likely to cause upset on both sides with little benefit for either patient or doctor.

Costs

The NHS was designed as a medical service which was free at the point of contact, the interface between the doctor and the patient. While that still holds true there have been changes to the funding of health care which are perceived as a potential source of conflict. Fundholding practices are allocated a budget with which to buy the bulk of their secondary-care services. The system does empower those practices which are fundholding and allows them to negotiate directly with secondary-care providers for services to their patients. However, the practice must work within a budget and it is theoretically possible for a practice to run out of funds in one financial year and have to defer referral to secondary care. Whose case should be deferred, what problem can wait? These decisions have the potential to change the role of the doctor from patient's advocate to financial arbiter.

Problems exist within secondary care at the time of writing over funding procedures and waiting lists. The local Health Authority holds the budget for patients who attend non-fundholding practices. Unfortunately they also have to meet the bills for accident and emergency departments and lengthy waiting lists have developed when funds will no longer stretch to include routine procedures. Although the situation is outside the control of the GP, it may be the GP who has to deal with the resulting frustrations to patient and family.

Resolving conflict with patients

We do not live or work in a perfect world where all patients, staff and doctors behave exactly as we would wish. We are, after all, only human. Systems and procedures do go wrong, communication breaks down occasionally and patients are disappointed when their expectations are not met. At their best our practice teams are caring, courteous, reasonable and efficient; at their worst, they are rude, abrupt, lacking in empathy and put administrative obstacles in the path of patients' needs.

In retailing the adage 'the customer is always right' is well known. Of course, it is not always true, but the onus is on the purveyor to make the customer feel valued. There is a parallel with patients, and we must endeavour at all times to make them feel valued by taking their views and comments seriously: like any customer they can seek an alternative supplier. Practices earn approximately 50 per cent of their NHS income from capitation payments. It is, therefore, imperative that they maintain a viable list size to survive, not only for capitation income but also for the potential to generate item of service income. Any patient who registers elsewhere in the same locality represents a failure to meet the desired level of service as well as a loss of income.

There will be times when a patient complains. In this section we will not try to distinguish between justified and unjustified complaints, but look at the process for handling a patient complaint in-house. If this part is dealt with correctly the likelihood of a complaint becoming a formal one will be minimised.

Patients' Charters

Many practices use a Patients' Charter to clarify exactly what a patient can, or cannot, expect from their practice. It is a document that should be publicised either by a poster in the waiting room or in an information folder in the waiting area, or both. The concept is simple – the practice clearly states the standards that they strive to maintain and those that they consider to be reasonable. A typical charter would include information about the following:

- practice leaflet;
- patient's right to general medical services;
- complaints procedures;
- repeat prescriptions;
- investigation results;
- confidentiality;
- waiting times to see the doctor;
- medical emergencies outside normal hours;
- access to medical records;
- booking appointments;
- arrangements for home visits;
- changes to systems.

Yet the benefit of writing such a document is felt more keenly by the practice team than by the patients. The process of systematically reviewing each service that the practice provides and then comparing it to the desired quality is educational. It also forces the primary health care team to put themselves in the consumer's position, rather than the customary provider one.

The charter targets must be realistic or two things will happen. The first will be an increase in patient complaints and the second will be the demotivation of the team. So any published aims should be totally realistic, even if they are not the standards that the practice ultimately aspires to. Each aim can be reviewed and raised, but it is much harder to lower them or consistently fail to meet them.

Example:

Appointments with a doctor:
- for routine consultations we will offer patients an appointment within two working days of the request.
- for medically urgent problems we will offer an appointment on the same day as the request.

This practice may have a longer-term ambition to see everyone on the same day as the request, but if the resources and systems are unavailable it would be incorrect to write it in their charter.

The Patients' Charter will also offer an opportunity to audit routine organisational functions. For example, if the charter states that all patients will be seen within 30 minutes of their booked appointment time how can we tell if this is actually happening? Audits are not just a vehicle for uncovering poor performance, they are intended to confirm the things that are done well too. To survey the length of time that patients wait to see the doctor may bring unexpected results.

Example:

The practice manager monitored the patients' booked appointment times against the times that the patient was called into the doctor's consulting room. At the end of morning surgery each doctor was late by the exact amount of time that the patients had arrived late!

This practice then embarked upon a patient-education campaign to stress the importance of arriving on time for their booked appointments.

A Patients' Charter is a form of patient education as it can help to convey the ways that patients can obtain the best service from their practice, and why certain demands are unlikely to be met. For example, if the Charter states that doctor's certificates and statements need to be handed in seven days before they are completed it will help to prevent a patient bringing in their passport application and photograph for signature and expecting to collect it an hour later.

The major criticism of charters by the medical profession has been that the document is totally biased by the needs of the patients with no regard to the needs of the doctors.

In fact, certain practices produced a Doctors' Charter at the same time as their Patients' Charter. This is unnecessary if the practice produces a balanced document giving reasons for particular issues.

The angry patient at reception

Few patients arrive angry; usually they come into the reception area with what they feel is a reasonable request. It is when those requests are not met with the expected reply that tempers flare. Earlier in this chapter we discussed the physical aspects of ambience and layout to avoid conflict with patients, but these measures are not infallible.

When a patient is causing a scene the first step should always be to defuse the situation by moving them to a quiet and private area. For this reason it is unwise to leave one person alone at the reception desk. A second person can either deal with the patient themselves or call for the assistance of the practice manager or a partner. There are times when to deal with a patient alone would be unwise, and personal security is dealt with later.

> I remember a patient who had a psychiatric problem and had spent some time in prison for attempted murder. His favourite phrase was, 'Am I mad or am I bad?' He developed a routine of wanting to see a doctor whenever his DSS payment was late, and became violent when the practice could not help. It seemed expedient to ensure that he was never left alone with just one member of the practice team! He was re-allocated regularly between the local surgeries and seemed to thrive on his own reputation.

The physical action of moving people away from the reception desk has several effects. Firstly, it reduces the level of embarrassment of all concerned, including other patients witnessing the exchange. Secondly, moving the angry patient into an environment where they have someone listening sympathetically to them acts as a calming force.

The knee-jerk reaction to a patient criticising the practice as a whole or an individual colleague is to become defensive and justify their actions. This simply generates more confrontation and will make matters worse. It is better to allow the patient to let off steam, then, when they are less emotional, start asking questions to establish the sequence of events and the specific nature of the complaint.

The other issue to consider is the most appropriate person to deal with a complaint, and a practice needs to be flexible in its approach. If the complaint is about a receptionist, then someone from a different area should deal with the patient. Often the practice manager is responsible for handling complaints, but there should be a back-up in case they are themselves the subject of the complaint.

The Complaints Procedure

In April 1996 a new NHS complaints procedure was introduced to make the handling of patient complaints a quicker and less threatening process for all parties. It was also intended to differentiate between investigations of a patient complaint and any subsequent disciplinary action deemed appropriate by the Health Authority.

The NHS Executive has produced a guidance booklet entitled 'Practice-based Complaints Procedures' which gives full details and explanations, as well as models for letters, notices and record forms. It is clearly written and every practice should ensure that the whole primary health care team are acquainted with the content and their responsibilities. There are some nationally-agreed criteria that all practices must adhere to:

- The complaints procedure must be 'owned' by the practice. In other words, every team member must understand the importance of resolving patient complaints quickly and efficiently and that no one is excluded from the guidelines. It is an essential part of a new employee's induction training.

  The Health Authority will only become involved if the practice system does not meet the national criteria, or at the request of the practice. They may require statistical data about numbers of complaints, but the details remain confidential to the practice.

- Every practice should nominate a person to administer the complaints procedure, and a deputy to cover in their absence.

- The existence and format of the practice complaints procedure must be made public via a waiting-room poster and written information that is freely available to patients.

- The written information should make it clear how to make a complaint:

  to whom?
  ↓
  what will happen after the initial contact?
  ↓
  who will contact them?
  ↓
  how long will it take?
  ↓
  possible outcomes

  It should also include details of how to access the health authority complaints procedure.

Keeping accurate records is vital, not only to ensure that the complaints administrator fulfills promises to write or telephone but also in case the complainant seeks help from the Health Authority. In this case, the Health Authority would need information about any action the practice has taken. It is advisable to maintain a specific complaints file and not to file copies of letters in the patient's medical records.

If a complaint is not resolved satisfactorily using the in-house procedure it may progress to include the Health Authority, and this is known as an Independent Review. As in general practice, the Health Authority will have a senior person with responsibility for patient complaints. They work closely with a Convenor, who is a non-executive director of the Health Authority, and who will examine each complaint and decide if it is appropriate for an Independent Review. The process can also include an independent lay person nominated by the Secretary of State for Health from a list held by the Regional Office of the NHS Executive. Should clinical advice be needed it is provided by general practitioners nominated by Local Medical Committees and based outside the Health Authority's area.

If an Independent Review is established, the panel will consist of three members, namely an independent lay Chairperson, the Convenor and an independent lay member. This panel has no disciplinary role, which is a change from the previous service committee hearings. The panel have the flexibility to decide the best way to handle each situation and report back to the complainant and practice, which may include comments about service improvements. A copy is sent to the Health Authority but this does not encompass recommendations about disciplinary action, which is for the Health Authority to decide.

The majority of complaints are resolved via the practice complaints procedure or an Independent Review. Should the complainant remain dissatisfied he or she can approach the Ombudsman or Health Service Commissioner. Simply going to the Ombudsman will not result in an automatic investigation; each case is considered prior to any action.

The effects of a complaint

Receiving a complaint about one's personal action, attitude or judgement is very distressing. It undermines confidence and can lead to endless re-examination of a particular sequence of events or situation. It is extremely difficult to view a complaint objectively and positively, especially if it is unfair or unfounded. In these situations our colleagues need support, and if the complaint is justified, help, to prevent a recurrence by counselling or training.

To minimise the anxiety of the person about whom the complaint is made, they should be advised as early as possible that a complaint has been received and invited to give their views of what happened. They should also be informed about the progress of the complaint through the practice-based procedure until a conclusion is reached. The temptation is to withhold information that might be upsetting, but this is a short-term gain and the issues will still need to be tackled at some point in time. Even if the member of staff or doctor was not at fault, they will need reassurance.

The positive side to patient complaints

There are many ways to seek patient feedback on the services offered and general organisational effectiveness of a practice. There may be a suggestion box, comment book and questionnaires in the reception area, all inviting patients to share their ideas and opinions. Most practices which have tried these types of initiative often discover that they are ignored, which signals that patients are happy with their lot or resigned to poor service. There is no substitute for hearing an angry or disillusioned patient's view of a specific incident. It provides the practice with meaningful, if slightly uncomfortable, evaluation of their systems and personnel.

It takes a great deal for the average patient to complain. General practitioners may have lost their place on top of a pedestal but they still enjoy a strong sense of loyalty from their patients, who are all too ready to tolerate, and even justify, the occasional failing or breakdown in communication. Therefore, to complain is a major event to a patient. We must take them seriously and use their comments to review systems constructively. The patient may have genuine concerns that a complaint may be held against them and that their medical care may suffer, so they perceive complaining as a high risk.

Remember, in industry it is accepted that for every person who complains another twenty stay silent but take their custom elsewhere. Monitoring the numbers of patients who register with another local doctor could be a revealing comment on the reputation of the practice.

Consequences of conflict

Consequences of conflict within the consultation can range from annoyance to catastrophe for either patient or doctor, or both. The failed relationship can cause frustration, anger and feelings of inadequacy in both parties with the doctor often blaming the patient for the situation; patients are often labelled as difficult or as troublemakers, possibly quite unjustly. Additionally, the difficult doctor–patient relationship has been shown to be associated with two to three times more tests, X-rays and referrals.

Litigation is on the increase and a difficult doctor–patient relationship is thought to be responsible for a significant proportion of cases. An angry or dissatisfied patient is thought to be as strong a motivator as actual negligence on the part of a doctor in making a complaint.

Verbal or physical aggression can be a consequence of conflict. Verbal aggression can come from just about anyone and as previously mentioned is the end result of a failed doctor–patient relationship with consequent failed communication, misunderstandings and misinterpretation. If it is not defused it can lead to physical aggression.

DEALING WITH AGGRESSION AND VIOLENCE

Physical aggression is increasingly mentioned in the medical press and the national media. During their working lives, most general practitioners will experience concerns for their safety at work. Some will have regular fears of aggression or violence, some will only experience such fears occasionally. There is not a lot of good information on the incidence of violence and aggression in general practice but the consensus is that it is increasing. What we see may only be the tip of the iceberg, as incidents may not be reported because of fear of retribution or because the victims seek to avoid publicity.

A survey of general practitioners in the West Midlands, done in 1989, while having limitations, produced some interesting data. The majority of incidents reported occurred within the consulting room and usually involved verbal abuse. Only 3 per cent of incidents involved violence. The situation changes when looking at the data for home visits. Violence, as you might expect, was more likely to occur during a domiciliary visit with serious violence being more likely during the quiet hours.

Two-thirds of aggressors were male; they were usually the patient or a relative and the vast majority were under 40 years of age. Very few incidents were caused by members of the general public and of those that were reported the vast majority were cases of verbal abuse. The survey looked at those involved and found that, as might be expected, drugs, alcohol, and anxiety, especially if compounded by a long wait or a bereavement and mental illness were leading precipitating factors. Of these mental illness was a significant factor for serious incidents of assault and injury.

Precipitating factors
- drug use
- alcohol use
- anxiety
- mental illness

The general practitioners involved in the study reported a number of changes to the way they practised. Unfortunately some of these reactions were counter-productive. Removing patients from your list does not really solve the problem, it merely transfers it down the road. Deputising services may relieve you of the immediacy of the problem but may change the balance of out-of-hours work and alter patient expectations. Unfortunately

---
- removing patient from list
- panic buttons
- increased use of deputising
- screens on reception
- increased police call-outs
---

although some general practitioners chose to install screens at reception there is evidence that these can actually increase incidence of aggressive incidents.

A number of personal effects were also reported. The doctors involved felt less committed to medicine and felt less confident when dealing with patients. They felt unable to visit in some areas and would prescribe, on demand, to angry patients. They felt very stressed by aggression and felt very intimidated by night calls.

The survey, although not necessarily generalisable and with a poor response rate, does give us some help when looking at ways we can structure our practices to prevent or deal with incidents if they occur.

Dealing with aggression is a team issue as any members of the team could be involved in an incident. Planning ahead is important and ideally your practice should have guidelines or protocols in place for use should an incident happen. We know that patients are more likely to be physically violent if they do not have the language skills or intellect to express their concerns and frustrations. Additionally, they often come from an environment where disputes are settled with violence. The survey gives us some indication of other at-risk groups – drug users, alcohol abusers the anxious, and mentally ill. With this information we can identify those at risk and can plan ahead.

Once at-risk patients have been identified, the system can be adapted to avoid other aggravating factors such as a long wait to see the doctor. Reception staff need guidance in how to handle a shouting patient and when to call the police. These guidelines should be constructed and agreed by the whole team using expert resources, such as the police, if necessary. Other members of the team must know that they are supported and that, to prevent escalation of a problem, they can interrupt a consultation. This may prevent aggression escalating to become violence.

When called to deal with an aggressive patient you must be careful. When you know you are in the right it is very tempting to say so, however, when faced with an aggressive patient your aim must be to stop the aggression escalating out of control and becoming physical violence. Confrontation is not a good idea and no attempts should be made to resolve any dispute while emotions are heightened. Use your body language to defuse the situation, be calm, keep a reasonable distance between you and the patient, keep your hands open and not folded across your chest or in fists. In keeping calm try not to move around too abruptly, do not frown and try and keep your jaw relaxed. Do not try to outstare the patient but maintain comfortable and non-threatening eye contact. Talk clearly but do not try to out-volume your patient!

Body Language
Keep calm
Keep a reasonable distance away
Keep hands down and relaxed
Keep brow and jaw relaxed
Keep comfortable but non-threatening eye contact

If the patient is very emotional it may be possible to try and calm him or her down perhaps by offering space and quiet, by acknowledging their grievance and if appropriate by apologising for any mistake however small. Often offering a cup of tea will act as a distraction and allow pause for thought. When dealing with the situation you must remain calm and cool. Calming thoughts or regular deep breathing as well as consciously not adopting an aggressive posture will help.

When faced with a violent patient your priority must be self-preservation. The aim is to avoid danger, not to right any perceived wrongs. Try and defuse the situation by adopting the body language and behaviours previously mentioned, appear confident but non-confrontational. Divert the patient from the situation if possible and swallow your pride. Look around for any ways of escape or for people who might be able to assist you. Remember they may be overwhelmed by the situation and will need your instructions to follow. Your first response may be indignation and anger but it is important that you release these emotions and act to preserve yourself from injury.

The aftermath of an incident must also be addressed. Being a victim is very unpleasant and upsetting and the upset may seem out of all proportion to the severity of the incident. Being a victim results in loss of self esteem and feelings of inadequacy. Those so traumatised need help. They need to talk through their experience and their feelings, preferably with someone who is trained appropriately.

The patient should be followed up as well. If the incident is severe there may be no alternative to removing him or her from the list. If it is less severe and with an understandable precipitant a discussion of the circumstances and the negotiation of future behaviour may be useful. In slow time, once the acute situation has resolved, you can explore the patient's concerns and discover the issues behind his or her behaviour. A calm discussion can then be held on why aggressive behaviour is unacceptable and a statement made that it will not be tolerated in the future. The ultimate sanction is, of course, removal from the list.

PRACTICE AND PERSONAL SECURITY

This is not an expert treatise on security but some general advice. Before undertaking any major expenditure we would recommend you undertake further research. In particular, if you wish to install alarms or panic buttons you would be well advised to seek the advice of your local security expert or crime prevention officer.

The practice

It is the duty of any employer to provide a safe and acceptable working environment. Part of that safety involves taking the appropriate security measures for your level of risk. You should be insured against an assault on yourself or your staff. You should regularly review your protocols, strategies and premises.

When reviewing your premises look at your reception area and waiting room. Ideally your reception should have deep, open-plan counters with perhaps a raised platform on the receptionists' side. Screened counters may actually increase the incidence of aggressive encounters. The waiting room should be a pleasant, comfortable area with toys and magazines as appropriate. The consulting rooms should also be pleasant areas laid out in a non-confrontational style. Resources can be found to help with improvements particularly if you practice in a high-risk area.

Training in the use of your protocols is essential. As there is some evidence that good communicators experience less violence than poor communicators, training in communication skills may be useful.

Personal security

There are a number of commonsense precautions which you should consider if you feel you may be put at risk. In the medical centre, never allow yourself to be alone with a potentially aggressive patient. Always have someone else in the building or nearby. Always have an escape route from a room, and if you suspect trouble keep yourself between the patient and the exit. For those going on a visit in a high-risk area, especially at night, there are a number of suggestions in Box 3.3.

Box 3.3

DON'T	*DO*
<ul><li>dress up, dress down</li><li>carry a doctor's bag</li><li>have loose hair – tie it back</li><li>wear high heels – you may have to run</li><li>allow the patient to block the exit</li><li>sit down – stay ready to move</li></ul>	<ul><li>tell someone where you are going</li><li>if possible take someone with you</li><li>have a mobile phone to hand</li><li>use a knapsack to carry kit – hands free</li><li>carry a torch</li><li>carry a personal alarm</li></ul>

Some doctors feel the need to take self-defence classes and if you work in a high-risk area that may boost your confidence. The concern is that you may become over-confident and try to cope with situations that you should run from.

HOW TO USE THE CONSULTATION AS LEARNING TOOL

A useful skill to acquire is the development of a consultation style which will allow you to minimise the incidence of conflict within the consultation. There are a number of well-known consultation models, which are described in separate texts. Each has elements which will prove useful in learning to identify and to manage conflict.

Some of the earliest workers on the consultation, Byrne and Long (1976), found that the most frequent reason for a consultation to be dysfunctional was that the doctor had not discovered the reason for the patient's attendance. This was supported by David Tuckett's (1985) work which also showed that patients' ideas, expectations and opinions were a sadly neglected resource within the consultation. Failure to look at these areas has already been mentioned as a potential cause of conflict. Consultation models today address these issues and you are well advised to use one or all of the models available to review your own consultations.

For example, Pendleton's *The Consultation* (Pendleton, Scofield, Tate and Havelock, 1990) describes a task-oriented model in which the consultation consists of seven tasks. Task one asks us to define the reason for the patient's attendance. Naturally if we do not find out what he or she has come for we are likely to fail

> **Task One**
>
> To define the reason for the patient's attendance, including:
> – the nature and history of the problems;
> – their aetiology;
> – the patient's, ideas and expectations;
> – the effects of the problem.

to satisfy his or her needs. Roger Neighbour in his *Inner Consultation* (1992) also has a schema for describing what goes on in the consultation and his first phase is called 'connecting'. In this phase a rapport is built up between the patient and the doctor, a rapport which is essential if the consultation is to address the patient's problem. Forming that rapport requires the doctor to develop both listening and observational skills. Both skills are necessary if you are to avoid conflict within your consultations.

Box 3.4

Task 2 – to consider other problems
Task 3 – with the patient to choose an appropriate action for each problem
Task 4 – to achieve a shared understanding of the problems with the patient
Task 5 – to involve the patient in the management and encourage him to accept appropriate responsibility
Task 6 – to use time and resources appropriately
Task 7 – to establish/maintain a relationship with the patient which helps to achieve the other tasks

Pendleton (1990) continues by looking at additional tasks which are listed in Box 3.4. The list is perhaps rather daunting but the book details a method of looking at videotaped consultations and eliciting the level at which each task is completed. Once you overcome the discomfort of watching yourself on video this is an excellent learning aid. Your own consultations can therefore be used to review behaviour and to look for ways that your manner and skills can be enhanced.

Roger Neighbour's model describes five phases the first of which, *connecting*, has already been discussed. The other phases are *summarising, handing over, safety netting* and *housekeeping*. The list for this model is not so daunting and is more easily remembered. Again the video proves a useful tool in discovering whether you too demonstrate these phases in your consulting.

SUMMARY

There are many issues that have to be considered when trying to minimise conflict within the consultation. We believe that we have discussed most of the important issues and would commend to you some of the texts mentioned in the reference list should you wish to explore some areas further. The most important thing to do however is to increase your awareness of the issues surrounding conflict and bring them to mind when you are next in a conflict situation.

REFERENCES

Berne Eric 1964 Games People Play. Penguin
Byrne P S & Long B E L 1978 Doctors Talking to Patients. HMSO
Helman Cecil 1990 Culture, Belief and Illness. Butterworth Heinemann
Hobbs F D R. 1994 'Aggression towards General Practitioners' in Wilkes T Violence and Health Care Professionals. Chapman and Hall
Liao K L 1994 'Violence in General Practice'. Pulse June 11 1994
Neighbour Roger 1992 The Inner Consultation. Kluwer
Payer L 1990 Medicine and Culture. Victor Gollancz
Pendleton D, Scofield T, Tate P, Havelock P 1990 The Consultation: an Approach to Learning and Teaching. Oxford Medical Publications
Schwenk T L & Romano S E 1992 'Managing the difficult Physician Patient Relationship'. American Family Physician Nov 1992
Tuckett D et al 1985 Meetings between Experts. Tavistock Publications

4. Conflict with staff

Most managers and partners would admit that they find problems with staff the most worrying part of general practice: employment legislation can be a minefield and some partnerships are unaware of their responsibilities as employers and the legal rights of employees. Every year we see more and more added to the statute books and managers need to keep themselves up to date if they are to manage their teams within the given guidelines. One of the latest pieces of legislation is the Disablement Discrimination Act, which has implications for the recruitment process as well as for employees who become disabled during their employment. The cost of contravening this and similar legislation is high. It could result in an industrial tribunal, which is distressing, time consuming and potentially expensive if the employer is found to have acted unfairly.

The practice which treats its team of staff fairly and with consideration and respect has no real fear of being sued for unfair dismissal, but prevention is infinitely better than cure.

In this chapter we will review the common staff problems and offer some techniques and examples of good practice to overcome them.

ATMOSPHERE AND ETHOS

The impact of partners

Few doctors appreciate the impact that their personal behaviour and attitude has on the rest of the team. Every nuance, comment and grumble is noticed and becomes the basis for general debate. Conversations between partners get overheard and are repeated, especially if comments refer to other partners or team members. The dangers of this are obvious – snippets of dialogue and indiscreet remarks generate inaccurate rumours and unnecessary speculation.

Good practice:

Partners should be encouraged to take their breaks together in a room where their conversations are not in the hearing of the general staff.

It is also possible for partners to get a totally wrong impression of their practice and the way it functions administratively. Many doctors arrive in the morning and start their surgery almost immediately. When they finish consulting there are home visits, prescriptions to be signed, telephone calls to return and queries to answer. They leave the building to do their visits, possibly attend a lunch-time meeting and return in time to commence their afternoon clinic or surgery. Inevitably a doctor gets only a brief series of snapshots of the team's workload. It is because partners' routines are pre-determined by appointment books and diaries that staff can use this information to show themselves in the best light. Impressions about the pressure of work can be distorted, either exaggerated or minimised. By late morning the frenetic telephone activity is largely over, requests for home visits have been received and allocated and the general feeling is one of relief that the worst of the day is over. If a partner regularly comes into the reception area at this point he or she may form the opinion that the practice is over-staffed. If this is verbalised the reaction will be one of disbelief and defensiveness, staff may manufacture work to do very visibly when that partner is in the vicinity and, at worst, a rumour may circulare that someone is going to be sacked.

Good practice:

If a partner has a comment about staffing levels it should be directed to the practice manager or raised at a partnership meeting, never voiced to the staff.

The staff are very skilled at picking up disagreements between partners, and the more manipulative will use it as an opportunity to pursue their own personal agenda. If it becomes obvious that the partnership is divided over a major issue, like fundholding or workloads, then this will be mirrored by staff. They will be quick to make their own views known to like-minded partners, often passing comments from the opposing camp. Normal interactions become distorted, everyone is watchful of the partners' behaviour and the atmosphere gets increasingly tense and uncomfortable.

Good practice:

When sensitive issues are under discussion the partners should agree a 'party line' that they can all maintain publicly.

Manipulative staff may also play the partners off against each other and the practice manager and they will be aware of each person's particular interests and preferences. They will have decided who, in the senior team, is most sympathetic to staff and perceived to be the most appreciative of their contribution. It is to this particular partner that they will take requests for new equipment, uniforms, salary increases and so on, in the hopes that the partner will champion their cause. Whilst the partner may feel flattered by having the staff's trust and confidence, there is a down side. His or her approachability and empathy may also attract additional work and queries. A late request for an urgent consultation or home visit is always a problem. The staff are only human and will choose the path of least resistance, that is, the partner who is most likely to agree without being difficult. Too often partners refuse such requests, implying that the member of staff is at fault for passing on a patient's dilemma and agreeing that it needs the personal attention of a doctor. 'Difficult' doctors soon generate a reputation for not understanding their team's responsibilities and the pressures they are under when dealing with patients. To avoid a barrage of grumbles or non-co-operation the staff become less amenable to patients and so fuel the 'dragon' image.

Good practice:

Strict guidelines for the distribution of appointments, extras and home visits should be agreed and adhered to by all parties. If the nominated partner cannot take the request they should liaise directly with a colleague – not pass it back to the receptionist.

The role of the manager

The practice manager's role in creating a harmonious working atmosphere is critical. He or she needs to gain a thorough knowledge of each team member and tackle the issues described above. A strong manager will participate in the formulation of practice policies, translate them into clear written guidelines, monitor the outcomes and support the staff in their execution. To be effective they must be seen to act fairly, including a willingness to deal personally with those who do not conform to agreed policies. Too often practice managers complain that they are neither partner nor staff, but in these situations it can be a positive advantage. The objectivity afforded by their position in the hierarchy allows them to maintain the needs and principles of the whole team as their sole aim.

Practice managers tend to come via three main routes, working their way up through the practice team, being recruited directly from a commercial background or transferring within the NHS. There is no doubt that establishing professional working relationships is hardest for those who have functioned at a different level within the practice. The ex-secretary will always be expected to type that urgent letter in a crisis, the ex-receptionist will be expected to cover the reception desk when regular staff are absent and the ex-computer secretary to help with a rush of repeat prescription requests. The transition from colleague to boss can be traumatic and the support of the partners is essential if the new manager is to develop fully into the role. Fortunately there are a number of professional bodies that a manager can join, namely the Institute of Health Services Management (IHSM), the Association of Managers in General Practice (AMGP) and the Association of Medical Secretaries Practice Administrators and Receptionists (AMSPAR). All of these organisations endorse training programmes that may result in a Certificate or Diploma in Management, linked directly to national standards (National Vocational Qualifications). Many managers find that their personal confidence and management skills are boosted by these courses and qualifications. Some of the conflicts that can arise between the manager and partners are covered in more detail in Chapter 6.

The decision-making team

The core decision-making team, usually the partners and practice manager, must send clear messages to the team and uphold them by their personal attitude and behaviour. If the partners consistently put the needs of the patients and the delivery of good clinical care above all else, so will the staff. Mixed messages, e.g. a written policy statement that patients who insist that they must be seen the same day will be given an emergency appointment at the end of morning surgery, but a Dr X who refuses to see any extras, will cause confusion and bad feeling. The staff will feel let down when they are only following the correct instructions.

A dysfunctional partnership team will generate a dysfunctional practice team. This does not mean that they must agree all the time over every issue; in fact, this would make matters worse. Every team goes through various stages of development and the model devised by Tuckman in 1965 is as relevant today as it was then. He describes the stages of team development as 'forming, storming, norming and performing'.

Forming

We can all remember being the newest person to join an established team. Irrespective of our title or position of authority, our reactions and emotions are the same. The driving force is our need to belong, be accepted and gain the approval of our new colleagues; for this reason we are watchful and anxious to conform the existing rules. This could be as simple as a dress code or as complicated as the corporate response to external bodies. We keep our personal views and feelings hidden and concentrate on getting acquainted with other members of the team. Part of this process is an assessment of the power base and we do our utmost to create a good impression with key people.

Storming

As a result of routine contact and shared experiences within the workplace our barriers begin to drop and we allow ourselves to expose more of our personal views. In brief, we become more relaxed in the company of colleagues. At this stage the likelihood of conflict is greatest, with inter-departmental squabbles and polarised opinions. A natural pecking order emerges as well as a desire to clarify everyone's role and responsibilities. Differing viewpoints become clear and, to develop, the group needs to respect these without feeling threatened.

Norming

The team that reaches this stage will begin to care about the collective performance. In general practice this would be, for example, concern about reputation and public image. Each team member recognises his or her own strengths and weaknesses, and those of colleagues. This allows for recognition of each person's limitations, which in turn makes for better delegation and task allocation. The team learns together from shared experiences and most conflicts have been resolved. The power struggles decline in importance as does the self-satisfaction of each individual.

Performing

To be totally effective every team should aim to reach this stage of development. The main characteristics include established relationships and improved communication. Everyone has a clear role, defined responsibility and authority, and familiarity with other personalities, and this facilitates direct and honest dialogue. The group's accepted standards maintain discipline and the team becomes self-regulating. Peer pressure is as powerful as imposed management censure. As the team matures the conflicts over power disappear, and the informal leadership moves from member to member according to the needs of the moment and the available skills.

From this analysis of team development it makes the impact of a new person easier to understand. Everyone moves back temporarily to the 'forming' stage and has to progress afresh. The more senior a new person, for example, a partner, the longer it will take for the team to regain its original level of performance.

Good practice:

Every new member of the team, including partners, should have an induction period and a nominated mentor to whom they can address queries and questions.

'Success breeds success' may be a hackneyed phrase, but the difference in atmosphere between a general practice consistently achieving high standards of service and clinical care and a low-achieving one is almost tangible.

CLEAR LEADERSHIP

We can all reflect on great leaders and attribute certain personal qualities to them. It may be drive, vision, decisiveness or charisma. Yet in general practice, apart from the single-handed practitioner, we must define corporate leadership. Earlier in the chapter we described the importance of clear messages, but how do we decide which message is the right one?

Dr Meredith Belbin (1981) devised various roles that need to be present in a successful team, based on an extensive period of research and observation. Each individual is a mixture of the given roles with a few clear strengths and a similar number of weaknesses. There is no 'right' or 'wrong' as every category needs to be present in a balanced and successful team. These are briefly described in Box 4.1.

Box 4.1

Team role	Positive Qualities
Company Worker	Organising ability, practical commonsense, hard-working, self-disciplined.
Chairperson	A capacity for treating and welcoming all potential contributors on their merits and without prejudice. A strong sense of objectives.
Shaper	Drive and a readiness to challenge inertia, ineffectiveness, complacency or self-deception.
Plant	Genius, imagination, intellect, knowledge.
Resource Investigator	A capacity for contacting people and exploring anything new. An ability to respond to challenges.
Monitor Evaluator	Judgment, discretion, hard-headedness.
Team Worker	An ability to respond to people and situations, promote team spirit.
Completer Finisher	A capacity for follow up. Perfectionism.

Interestingly there is no category for 'leader'. We can go though the positive qualities and pick out points from each team role that are desirable in a leader, hence if each team role is present within the partnership then the capability to lead must also be there. The challenge is to harness these qualities and translate them into something practical.

We cannot lead without a clear aim or if we have no means of measuring if we have achieved anything worthwhile. In the early 1990s it was the vogue to have a mission statement, and many Family Health Services Authorities (now Health Authorities or Boards) were offering funding and facilitation for practices who wished to have one. They are not as popular now, but the importance of having a clear aim has not diminished. The usual mission statement for a general practice was along the lines of, '*To deliver a high standard of care that is readily accessible and available to all our patients*'. To be relevant to the whole primary health care team there should be several subsidiary mission statements, one for each area of the organisation. For example, for the practice manager it might be, '*To be responsible for the efficient, effective and safe, administrative, personnel and financial management of the practice.*' Mission statements explain what is expected in broad terms, not how to achieve it. The same themes should permeate throughout the organisation to secure consistency.

The process of agreeing a mission statement can take longer than the resulting simplistic phrase suggests. It requires each member of the primary health care team to identify their professional priorities in all aspects of accessibility, clinical standards, audit, continuing education and so on. Some groups will find this straightforward if they are used to exchanging and comparing this type of information. For them it will be an uncomplicated exercise in ranking each topic and deciding the appropriate wording. The partnerships who do not regularly participate in this kind of debate may feel quite daunted at the prospect. It may expose fundamental differences, for example, if one partner sees generating more income as the sole priority and another wishes to invest in medical equipment to increase the range of patient services. These debates cannot be aired adequately within routine meetings; they will require time and research if a compromise is to be reached. For this reason many partnerships opt to go away from the practice for a day to have an undisturbed quality discussion.

Away days

The reaction to 'away days' is mixed. Some practices prevaricate for a great deal of time before agreeing to have one, possibly because the partners feel threatened by the potential exposure to criticism from their team or because they cannot see a positive outcome that will justify the expenditure. Yet, interestingly, once they have had one they are keen to repeat the exercise annually or bi-annually. Those practices who wish to organise such an event should contact their Health Authority for advice about partial funding and to seek recommendations for a facilitator. In its simplest terms, an 'away day' is an extended meeting for selected members of the team or the whole team. Any issue can be tackled, for example, building new premises, embarking on the additional responsibility of becoming a training practice, or a business planning session.

'Away days' are usually facilitated by suitably qualified person who can chair the discussions and workshops and who will 'manage' differences of opinion. A facilitator will allow every team member to participate fully, without the distraction of organisation and preparation. They should also ensure a balanced discussion and give everyone an equal opportunity to contribute. Their aim is to seek realistic agreements and objectives and to secure compliance for the future. Some practices take the whole team, some just the partners and practice manager, and some a small group comprising a representative from the main groups within the practice, e.g. receptionist, practice nurse, community nurse, secretary, etc. If the whole team is not invited some method must be found to inform them of the outcomes and gain their commitment. Otherwise the exercise will be totally wasted, as will a mission statement in name only. Many practices type their statements and post them in prominent positions around the practice. Again, this is a futile exercise if the practice does not uphold its published intentions.

Once the mission statements have been agreed they must be supported by specific objectives. The practical implications for the practice have to be identified, resources allocated and deadlines set for their achievement. Bearing in mind that there will be a range of short-term, medium-term and long-term objectives the workload should be fairly evenly spread.

Techniques

There are some simple techniques to analyse a practice and assist in planning. One of the common ones is a SWOT analysis (Box 4.2), another is a PESTLE analysis (Box 4.3). The former tends to be a stocktake of the internal and immediate situation, whereas the latter invites a wider look at how an individual organisation relates to the outside world.

Box 4.2

SWOT analysis	
<u>S</u>trengths	– knowing your strengths so that you can feel confident and capitalise on existing resources
<u>W</u>eaknesses	– knowing your weaknesses so that unwise decisions are avoided and a strategy can be planned to overcome them
<u>O</u>pportunities	– identifying new opportunities so that innovations can be injected into the organisation
<u>T</u>hreats	– detecting and anticipating threats so that defensive action can be taken in good time

The SWOT analysis is very flexible and can be used to analyse almost any situation.

Box 4.3

PESTLE analysis

POLITICAL
ECONOMIC
SOCIAL
TECHNOLOGICAL
LEGAL
ECOLOGICAL

An example of a PESTLE analysis on the National Health Service can be seen in Box 4.4.

Box 4.4   Example PESTLE analysis

Political
  – changes imposed by Government
  – de-regulation in White Papers
  – taxation (e.g. Employer's National Insurance)
  – education and training
  – monopolies and mergers (e.g. pharmaceutical companies)

Economic
  – accountability for NHS costs
  – grants and subsidies
  – the public sector

Social
  – demographic changes
    – decline in birth rate
    – increase in number of elderly
  – increased expectations
  – rise in cynicism
  – consumerism

Technological
  – the paperless practice
  – confidentiality
  – home working

Legal
  – health and safety
  – employment
  – industrial relations
  – accounting practices
  – product liability

Ecological
  – the 'green' revolution
  – animal testing

The benefits of undertaking this kind of analysis as a group are many and varied. The partners gain valuable input from all sectors of the team and hear different perspectives on perceived problems. It is an educational exercise as the whole team rarely get an opportunity to pool information. Internal and inter-departmental power struggles diminish as the staff's awareness of their contribution to the whole process of delivering quality primary care increases. Most importantly, barriers drop and a team approach develops. In this environment any decisions that are taken collectively have a high success rate.

FEELING VALUED

Most direct conflict with staff originates from their belief that they are not valued by their employers, the partners. This comprises a number of elements, for example, involvement in the decision-making process, being treated fairly, having a clear sense of purpose and direction, having equity of opportunity and being listened to when they have an innovative idea or grievance. If we can make the individual feel valued within the organisation we have a firm base upon which to build the team.

To understand how to make the individual feel valued we must first understand their basic needs. The difficulty is that we employ human beings, each with a different set of personal and professional objectives. A measure or policy that motivates one person does not necessarily have the same effect on another.

The work of Abraham Maslow (1970), exemplified in his Hierarchy of Basic Human Needs (Box 4.5), helps us to identify clear methods of appropriate reward and motivation.

Taking the first, and most important, physiological need of staff will lead us to look at the fundamental principles of employment – the salary structure. People need a reason to work and it is usually the improved lifestyle that they can afford with a regular income. For the only wage-earner in a household it may to used to cover basic living expenses, like food and heating. When the income is supplementary to another in the household the motivation may be the non-essential, but ego-boosting items, like holidays or a new car. Very few of us believe the statement, 'I don't need to work, I'm only looking for an interest and company'. If this were really the case the applicant would be seeking voluntary work! Irrespective of the reason, an individual will have decided before applying for a particular

Box 4.5   Maslow's Hierarchy of Human Needs

PHYSIOLOGICAL
e.g. food, water, temperature control
i.e. physical survival
↓
SAFETY
e.g. security, freedom from fear, the need for law, order,
structure and limits
↓
SOCIAL
e.g. love, affection, affiliation, acceptance by others
↓
ESTEEM
e.g prestige, status, self-respect and respect from others
↓
COGNITIVE
e.g. knowledge, understanding, curiosity
↓
AESTHETIC
e.g. beauty, art, symmetry
↓
SELF-FULFILMENT
e.g. achievement, realisation of potential

job what they will gain. This is beyond any employer's control and our job begins in the workplace.

Whilst salary is not the sole motivator, the overall policy must be fair. It should differentiate between levels of responsibility and skills, compare favourably with similar employers and be published in-house so that everyone sees clearly where they are in relation to colleagues. The Whitley Council is the commonly applied salary structure for general practice and, if used fairly, fulfils the criteria mentioned above. There are clear definitions of each level of responsibility and a progression to an upper limit that rewards long service. The problems arise when the scales are inappropriately applied or when an employee is given an hourly rate that falls outside the stipulated range. Conflict develops when an individual is paid a different rate to a colleague for performing the same role, or when additional responsibility and training does not attract an increase in salary. When this basic aspect is properly organised and implemented the needs of staff will move on to some of the other issues.

We are fortunate in general practice that we have a clear place in the community. Although the GPs' position on a pedestal may have been eroded, they still enjoy a positive reputation for being part of the caring profession. By association, the staff can share the reflected glory. This helps to address the social needs of the individual, which are enhanced by the working environment. We see many small indicators that this is happening, for example, cakes on special occasions, small kindnesses, visits to colleagues who are ill or in hospital and, more recently, lottery syndicates.

When faced with an imposed change our natural reaction is to rebel against it, yet if we are involved in the consultation process we would accept the same decision without demur. The practice that routinely and automatically includes staff and seeks their opinions about proposed change will experience fewer problems than one which does not. We are effectively paying due respect to the individual's knowledge and experience, and not falling into the trap of arrogance by assuming that we know better than those doing the job. This equates to 'esteem' on Maslow's hierarchy.

COMMUNICATION

High standards in communication are the key to avoiding conflict and they are implicit in every example of good practice. If the team has progressed to the 'performing' stage the characteristic communication will be open and honest, and constructive criticism will be a routine part of working life.

The common barometer of communication is the number of meetings that take place, but quality is as important as quantity. There must be a clear purpose to each meeting, with a demonstrable value. A typical practice would hold the meetings listed in Box 4.6, with varying regularity according to need.

Effective meetings

For all meetings there are tried and tested techniques that can improve their effectiveness.

Timing

Some meetings are doomed because they are called at inconvenient times for the participants. An example of this would be a partners' meeting arranged on a Monday morning, which is the busiest time of the week. The effect is likely to be a large number of apologies or

Box 4.6   Practice meetings

BUSINESS and POLICY
CLINICAL
EDUCATIONAL
STAFF
MANAGEMENT TEAM
SOCIAL
AWAY DAYS (strategic planning, problem solving)
SPECIAL PROJECTS (recruiting a partner, new premises)
PRIMARY HEALTH CARE TEAM
PURCHASING

doctors leaving early to see patients. The outcome is the same – decisions cannot be taken if the whole group is not present, or without a level of debate. If decisions are made the absent partner(s) may choose to exercise their power of veto and overturn them.

Agenda

It is unfair to expect a full and informed discussion about any topic without advance warning. An agenda is a crucial tool to prepare and maintain focus in a meeting. Ideally one person is nominated to collect agenda items from all parties and circulate the agenda well in advance. A good discipline is to ask those who place an issue on the agenda to also produce some supporting information to be circulated at the same time. This allows people time to think and minimises the risk of emotional reactions. Time management is improved if the estimated amount of time needed for each item can be judged and workload matched to time available more accurately.

Advance warning

The greater notice we can give to participants the more likely is it that they will attend. For regular meetings, e.g. monthly, it is useful to agree a pattern, e.g. the first Tuesday at 1.00 pm. This assists everyone in planning their diary and they are less likely to forget. Circulating the agenda acts as a useful reminder.

Chairing the meeting

The nomination of a chairperson is the most important decision in the meeting process. They have a number of responsibilities, for example, timekeeping, maintaining focussed discussion, ensuring everyone contributes, summarising points of view and pinpointing future actions. The chairperson is a facilitator rather than participant and chairing requires special skills, as well as the respect of the participants. The traditional right of the chairperson to have the casting vote means that they should not have a significant role in a persuasive discussion.

Follow-up

A record of all formal meetings should be made and circulated in the form of minutes. These have a dual purpose, firstly to tell people who could not attend what took place, and secondly to remind attendees of the decisions and discussions. Full minutes, that is, a summary of who said what, can be lengthy and in view of this may not be read. It is acceptable to re-design minutes to take the format of an 'action plan'. One side of A4 paper with easily digested bullet points is more likely to be read than a six-page document (Box 4.7). It may also make the participants realise how little was actually decided. Once committed to paper the decisions need to be followed through and the person that this duty should fall to is the chairperson.

Box 4.7   Example of an 'Action List'

MEETING HELD on 1st June		
Decision	Person Responsible	Deadline
To award a staff salary increase		
– to cost an increase of 3% for all staff		
– to cost an increase of 5% for all staff	Practice	
– to compare rates of pay with other local practices	Manager	1st July
– to agree final details at July meeting	All Partners	
– to be effective from 1st September		
To hold an 'Away Day' in November		
– to contact HA for suitable facilitators	PM	1st August
– to seek sponsorship from drug reps	Dr A.	1st August
– to find out information about a venue, including costings and available dates	PM	1st August
– to find a locum	PM	1st August
– to discuss further at August meeting including a date	All Partners	

Cascading information

Part of the decision-making process should be the way in which information is disclosed, and to whom. Some meetings, like ones that include all the staff, are straightforward. However, some partnership policy meetings have confidential issues that it is not appropriate to communicate to everyone. There is nothing more annoying to staff than to be told haphazardly about decisions that affect practice administration and organisation. If staff meetings can be linked to practice meetings, ideally taking place the following working day, then a uniformity can be achieved and the staff will have an opportunity to discuss the rationale behind any policy decision, the practical implications can be resolved and a date agreed for new methods to commence.

When practice decisions affect groups outside the practice, e.g. the community team, then a person should be nominated to liaise and explain (Box 4.8).

Box 4.8

Example:

Dr Green announces his intention to retire on 31st December at a practice meeting held on 1st June. The partners agree that they wish to replace Dr Green with a full-time partner to take over his list of 2000 patients.

Who needs to know?	How?	Person responsible
Practice team	Special staff meeting	Practice Manager and Dr Green
Attached staff	Individual letter	Dr Green
Patients	Letter from Health Authority when new partner appointed	Practice Manager and Health Authority
Consultants Local GPs Accountant Bank Manager Hospitals	Letter from practice when new partner is appointed	Practice Manager

---

Memos and letters

When we are short of time and need to circulate information quickly it is tempting to send a memo rather than talk to each individual.

The main drawback of a memo is that it can be seen as terse and impersonal. If the written word does not exactly match our sentiments then the wrong impression will be created. No one will worry about the wording of a memo that tells everyone they are getting a pay rise, but send a disciplinary memo and they will. A compromise would be a well-considered letter addressed to each individual, which also implies that the matter deserves their personal attention.

Protocols

There are situations when clear guidance is essential: one would be what to do if the fire-alarm sounds. In this instance we are not going to go to each member of staff and debate the merits of evacuating the building, instead we would sound the fire-alarm and expect immediate action. We saw a major influx of protocols in 1990 when health-promotion clinics were introduced as part of the new GP Contract. To qualify for payment each practice had to submit a written protocol for each clinic they wished to claim for. Since the health-promotion payments have changed most practices have taken a more rational view and maintain protocols for delegated clinical duties, for example, chronic-disease clinics and new-patient checks. They do have an application beyond the clinical into the organisational aspects of general practice, where a uniform approach is required. A typical reception desk protocol would be the way that appointments should be booked or how a telephone emergency should be handled. To keep a file containing all the protocols provides a useful source of reference as well as a training tool for new or relief staff.

Electronic communication

The introduction of fax machines and modem links has completely changed our options for sending data out of the practice. Not only is a one-page fax cheaper than a local telephone call, it is a better use of time. Information arrives instantly on the recipient's machine and we do not spend the first few minutes exchanging pleasantries as we do with a telephone conversation. The World Wide Web or Internet has given us the facility to link with other computer users via a modem and we send messages or E-mail from screen to screen. The main benefit to general practice of 'surfing the web' is the access to clinical information and research papers around the world.

There are now occasions when our patients have accessed such information and present it to their doctor for comment.

To date the issue of protecting confidentiality has not been fully explored in relation to the electronic transfer of data. We have all heard the horror stories of termination of pregnancy details being sent to the local bank, and, although rare, these things can happen. Some hospitals refuse to fax patient information, e.g. discharge summaries, and some practices ask the patient for their written permission to fax their medical details to a third party.

Whatever communication medium we use it must be appropriate for the purpose and desired outcome.

JOB DESCRIPTIONS AND CONTRACTS

Employers are obliged to issue every member of staff with a Contract of Employment and job description by the end of the second month of their employment.

Job descriptions

We have identified the need for clear aims earlier in this chapter and a job description is simply these objectives broken down into detail and attributed to each role within the team, i.e. the 'what to do'. Too often job descriptions are a list of tasks and responsibilities grouped under main headings, which has limited application. A more meaningful approach is to combine the 'what to do' with some measurable quality indicators, thereby setting clear standards which can be audited and reviewed (Box 4.9).

Box 4.9   Example of job description with measurable indicators

---

Dealing with telephone enquiries
- answer the enquiry line within four rings
- deal courteously with all calls
- transfer calls to the appropriate person to deal with the query if you are unable to resolve it
- keep the caller informed if you are unable to connect them immediately
- record all calls in the telephone log book

The responsibility is to deal with telephone enquiries, but this has been expanded to include standards that can be measured and monitored.

This principle is also used when designing Charter Standards, but too often we produce these kinds of documents because we have been instructed to do so by our administrative masters. This blinds us to the genuine raising of standards that a job description can offer. For established and experienced staff the introduction of a job description may seem rather superficial, but it can be turned into a motivational task if the individual is asked to write their own. This has a distinct advantage to the manager – it requires less time and will increase the manager's knowledge of the various tasks.

The job description is an essential document which has a number of valuable uses:

- initial training for new staff;
- remedial training;
- appraisal;
- setting measurable standards;
- developing practice ethos.

To refer back to Maslow's second human need, safety, a job description explains the parameters of the role and the required standard of performance. These factors combine to represent security, in that the individual's job is safe if they conform to expected levels. They also inspire confidence and trust in the employer by the increased awareness of the organisation's overall aims and the contribution that they, as an individual, can make.

Contracts

A contract of employment exists when an employer and an employee agree upon the terms and conditions of employment, and both parties are bound by the agreed terms. Any employee who works more than eight hours per week must be given a written contract.

The minimum content should be statements and details of the following:

- name and address of employer;
- name and address of employee;
- job title;
- place of work;
- rate and method of pay;
- hours of work;

- term of employment;
- holiday entitlement and holiday pay;
- sickness or injury;
- pensions;
- disciplinary procedures;
- grievance procedures;
- periods of notice.

Many practices have developed the minimum requirements of a contract into a booklet encompassing all the terms and conditions of employment. For members of the British Medical Association there are some excellent guidance notes available for non-medical staff. The DTI (Department of Trade and Industry) also produce a range of advisory booklets that are available free of charge from Job Centres and Citizens' Advice Bureaux.

The advantage of a comprehensive booklet is as a training guide for new staff and reinforcement for existing staff. It can include organisational systems, codes of conduct, general information, practice aims and objectives, training and confidentiality: in short, anything that the partnership expects from their staff.

The most sensitive part of employment is discipline. Few people enjoy the prospect of having to criticise a colleague formally or even informally. Yet not to do so can result in greater problems. For example, if a member of staff is repeatedly late and the manager appears to condone it because they ignore it, then the group standards suffer. Other staff may start being late and nothing can be said as the situation has gone too far. The only remaining course of action is to issue a general directive about punctuality which will upset the majority of the staff, when a simple cautionary word at the outset would have prevented the situation escalating.

A disciplinary procedure is essential as it provides clear terms of reference and secures equality of treatment. If the procedure is followed accurately it will allow the employer to discipline and even dismiss a member of staff fairly (Box 4.10).

Time invested at the beginning of the process to produce or develop staff contracts will avoid the type of crisis management that arises when a difficult situation occurs and there is no written guidance to clarify the desired standard of behaviour or performance.

Box 4.10   Example of a disciplinary procedure

ENQUIRY
Discussion about a complaint or criticism with the individual concerned.

↓

COUNSELLING
Help, advice and possibly further training will be offered to resolve the criticism.

↓

VERBAL WARNING
A formal meeting detailing the exact nature of the complaint and the required standard. Notice of the meeting will be given in writing and in advance. If it is appropriate at the end of this meeting a verbal warning will be given and confirmed in writing to the individual.

↓

WRITTEN WARNING
If the individual's behaviour or performance still causes concern a further meeting will be arranged, as before. The likely consequences of further poor performance or conduct will be explained and the individual given a period of time to improve. At the end of this meeting a formal written warning will be given to the individual.

↓

FINAL WRITTEN WARNING
Should the individual's performance or behaviour still not reach the required standard there will be a further disciplinary meeting. A written warning given at this stage will be a final written warning, and failure to improve may result in dismissal.

↓

DISMISSAL
Should the individual fail to meet the required standards a further disciplinary hearing will be arranged, as before. The notice of dismissal will include the appeal procedure.

↓

APPEAL
An appeal may be made against a final written warning or dismissal. Full written reasons for the appeal must be submitted within 14 days of receipt of the final written warning or written confirmation of dismissal.

TRAINING AND DEVELOPMENT

The importance of training for staff and doctors has been reinforced in recent years by the introduction of Postgraduate Education Allowances and staff-training budgets. We live and work in an ever-changing environment, and advances in technology and administration necessitate the constant updating or enhancing of skills and competencies. We cannot simply employ new people who possess the new skills and ignore longer-standing staff, we must help each individual to learn and progress. There are a number of ways to do this, some on a team basis and some on an individual one. This links back to the 'cognitive' and 'self-fulfillment' stages of Maslow's hierarchy of human needs.

Personal objectives

Earlier in the chapter we discussed the importance of setting clear aims and objectives, and various methods of producing them. To turn this from an academic exercise to a meaningful one the business objectives must be translated into personal ones.

All objectives, whether corporate or individual must be SMART.

S	–	Specific
M	–	Measurable
A	–	Achievable
R	–	Realistic
T	–	Timed

Imposing these criteria on any objective will guard against an unsatisfactory result. For example, rather than tackling one major objective in vague terms it is easier, and more effective, to break it down into smaller ones and allocate them between all members of the primary health care team.

Corporate objectives relate to personal ones as shown in Figure 4.1.

Appraisal

The word 'appraisal' can have threatening connotations for the recipient if the process is not handled correctly and sensitively. Many of us have images of school reports, a totally subjective judgment of performance and rigid marking. None of these could be considered motivating! A definition of appraisal would be '*a regular review which provides an opportunity to summarise past performance and plan for the future*'. Appraisal need not be formal or focus upon forms, it can be a relaxed and routine interaction with staff. The important point is that it happens regularly and gives each individual an

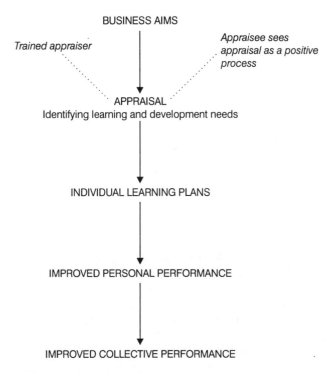

Figure 4.1

opportunity to air their views and receive feedback on their performance and contribution. Done well, appraisal benefits the individual, the manager and the organisation in the following ways:

The individual

- how is he/she getting on?
- hears views from others;
- discussion about personal contribution;
- future learning and development;
- understands how his/her role contributes to the whole team.

The manager

- gains the individual's view of his/her performance;
- mutually agrees strengths and weaknesses;
- identifies training and learning needs;
- obtains better knowledge of staff;
- generates ideas to benefit the organisation;
- gains feedback on his/her own performance as a manager.

The organisation

- closer working relationships;
- motivates staff;
- identifies potential and limitations of each individual;
- helps to plan for the future;
- encourages openness and honesty.

Appraisals do not just happen, they have to be carefully prepared. Each member of staff should get notification of the interview and, new staff especially should be given an outline of the format. This will assist each individual to think of the important issues that they wish to raise. Some practices write these points in a standard letter and some do it verbally.

The manager needs to get a balanced view of the individual's general performance and guard against bias from a 'one-off' event. This may involve other people within the practice, such as a senior receptionist or office manager. However, these fact-finding conversations must be kept strictly confidential and not disclosed to the individual concerned prior to the interview. The actual standard required is detailed in the job description and an annual review of this document may do one of two things: highlight how out of date it is or disclose certain tasks that the individual does not or cannot do.

The manager conducting the appraisal must also prepare thoroughly. If a form is not used then a list of points to cover is essential. It is useful to have both the job description and contract of employment to hand, as well as specific examples of any criticisms. The contract is helpful if the individual wishes to query things like holiday entitlement and salary structure. It is not only the appraisee who can feel threatened at the thought of an appraisal interview, the person conducting it can have similar reservations!

An appraisal interview has seven main stages:

- an overview of the practice aims;
- discussing the individual's current role;
- strengths and weaknesses;
- training and learning needs;
- agreed personal objectives;
- topics that the appraisee wishes to discuss;
- summary.

As in all confidential interviews any appraisal should take place in an undisturbed and comfortable environment, and be conducted with a person empowered and with sufficient knowledge to undertake a detailed analysis of responsibilities and workload. The appraiser should also have enough authority to ensure that all issues and promises are followed up.

All appraisal interviews start on a positive note just because the individual is given quality time to discuss themselves and their feelings. This can be easily destroyed and it is the skill of the interviewer that will prevent this happening. Most conversations within general practice take place 'on the hoof': we begin to discuss a system or problem only to get called away by telephones, patients or doctors.

There are some techniques that will help to overcome some of the difficulties in an appraisal interview. One has already been mentioned, namely that there should be specific examples of every criticism. It also helps to have a time plan for each stage to ensure that the interview does not become abrupt and is not curtailed unnecessarily, but equally that it does not last for too long and degenerate into a general chit-chat. Nothing should come as a surprise to the individual, and all comments should have been raised previously as part of routine discipline. Apart from offering an overview and explanations, the interviewer should do more listening than talking, and when they do speak use unambiguous language. We are all human and prefer some people to others, but in any formal interview we must keep personal feelings and emotions firmly hidden. The conversations should be on a factual level, and using evidence-based comments will avoid any temptation to show favouritism.

Finally, the appraisal gives us an opportunity to do something that employers are generally very bad at – say 'thank you' or 'well done'. Recognition of contribution by praising someone is a powerful, and the cheapest, motivator. To have this included in a written summary of the appraisal will do much for morale.

Delivering training

Most people, if asked, consider training to be something that happens away from the workplace at a special event. Appraisal can help to change this attitude by offering alternatives and developing the concept of the learning practice. Dr Peter Havelock has done a great deal of work in the old Oxford Region on this issue, and although it centres around GP vocational training practices it has many applications for every practice. Part of the process is the provision of educational opportunities, both clinical and organisational, and it requires everyone in the primary health care team to share their knowledge and skills.

The range of learning opportunities in every practice is very broad, and instead of being the poor relation, in-house teaching can be the most effective.

Why should we learn?

- to achieve and maintain the desired level of performance

- to develop each individual to attain their full potential

- to create a cost-effective team

- to motivate by encouraging a sense of belonging

- to increase job satisfaction by making the individual feel valued

- to prepare for future challenges

When we review what we learn it becomes apparent that a workplace setting is the most appropriate for, for example, information about practice policies, new systems and working methods, increased knowledge about the primary health care environment, initial training for new staff and the indoctrination of practice ethos and established standards. Very few learning needs, with the exception of personal development and specific skills, like word processing, are best undertaken away from the practice.

Outside courses

Outside courses should not substitute for what the practice can deliver, but be used sparingly to target specific learning and development needs. External courses are the most expensive medium and care should be taken before sending staff. The Health Authority should be able to offer guidance based on feedback from previous delegates; failing that, some research into the topics covered and the calibre of the tutor is essential.

External tutor

When the whole team has a general training need, e.g. handling complaints, it may be more viable to bring in a tutor to run a session. This has the advantage of being excellent value as the venue costs are minimal if the session is held in the practice, and per capita the costs will be low. This is the same principle as an away day, although the emphasis is shifted from a 'working together' day to a more technical learning day.

In-house

The training budget is not restricted to expenditure on outside courses and a well-planned and executed in-house scheme may be approved for reimbursement by the Health Authority. Too often the range of abilities that can be shared for the benefit of the whole practice is overlooked. For example, a Health Visitor is skilled with children on the 'at risk' register and can explain the surrounding legislation and responsibilities to doctors and administration staff.

In-house training happens in a number of ways:

- 'sitting with Nellie';
- formal tutorials;
- informal chats;
- situation analysis;
- meetings;
- reading;
- written protocols and memos;
- job swapping;
- disciplinary procedures;
- in-house presentations;
- training videos;
- networking.

Some practices dedicate an hour each week or fortnight for staff training and either close over a lunch-time or take half the team at a time to give adequate cover. Training should be seen as part of everyday working life, not a 'one off' that is in some way special. Systems that rely on goodwill and unpaid overtime, e.g. a session in the evening, are unlikely to be successful.

The perceived risk of training

One of the common obstacles to introducing an in-house programme or to sending a delegate to an expensive course is the view that staff will instantly leave and take their skills elsewhere for a higher salary. This perception is difficult to change and the benefits of a well-trained and competent team are hard to quantify. Much staff dissatisfaction and conflict comes from not feeling valued or from feeling that they are deliberately kept in the dark.

In conclusion, conflict with staff is usually avoidable. If the practice fosters and demonstrates a caring environment for patients that is naturally extended to staff and doctors it is more likely to be harmonious. The practice manager has a vital role in ensuring that their personal management skills are adequate and that they, in turn, can introduce strong personnel systems and maintain open channels of communication between all parties.

REFERENCES

Tuckman B W 1965 'Development sequences in small groups'. Psychological Bulletin, 63, pp384–399
Belbin R M 1981 Management Teams: why they succeed or fail. Heinemann, London
Maslow A H 1970 Motivation and Personality. 3e, Harper and Row, New York.
Hasler J C et al 1991 Handbook of Practice Management. Longman Group
Havelock P 1995 onwards The Learning Practice. Various lectures and presentations in the old Oxford Region where Dr Havelock is an Associate Adviser

5. Conflict with partners

When there are partnership difficulties they almost always revolve around workload, finance or the future direction of the practice. Not quite so common are concerns about a partner's performance, poor physical or mental health, alcohol or drug abuse or unsafe clinical practice. These are key issues where strong feelings are provoked and firm views held by individual partners. Occasionally the real reasons for conflict are concealed, and a lesser problem is used to bring it out into the open because a completely honest discussion would be painful for all parties. To tackle the root causes of partnership conflict takes great courage and hard evidence. To salvage a partnership after this type of experience takes much more courage, such as a willingness to grow and learn together and to establish new working relationships. There are times when differences are so overwhelming that a partnership split or resignation is the only option. The real test of a practice, and the relationships within it, comes when something starts going wrong and the perceived satisfaction of one or more of the partners changes. In this chapter we will explore the causes of partnership conflict, dealing with a partnership dissolution and sensible precautions to maintain a problem-solving mechanism. Throughout the text there will be examples of 'real life' to illustrate the sort of situations that can arise and their outcomes.

ORGANISATIONAL MODELS

The ability to overcome and harness conflict will depend upon the type and style of the organisation. Dr Richard Flew, an Associate Adviser in the old Oxford Region, has developed Dr Peter Havelock's work on the learning practice into organisational models to demonstrate a partnership's problem-solving capacity. They succinctly describe alternative partnership structures and the way each one reacts to an obstacle.

The cube

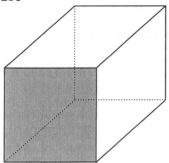

At first glance a cube would appear to be a suitable model for a practice. There are rigid lines for communication and reporting procedures implying structure and control. It will move easily on a slope, but has no natural energy of its own to move unaided by its environment. When it does move its shape will only allow it to move in a straight line or tip over on its side. If a cube meets an obstacle, like a brick wall, it will hit it with some force and may find that its corners get chipped or knocked off completely. If the obstacle is solid and the cube is moving at speed it may shatter and fragment.

The ball

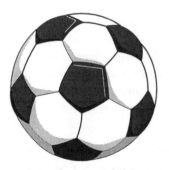

The ball seems to have some desirable characteristics that are not present in the cube. It is far more responsive and will quickly gather momentum if the surface upon which it rests tilts or slopes. The structure is not quite so rigid, but still retains a definite shape. The movement does not come from within, only from external influences.

However, when a ball hits an obstacle in its path it will bounce in an unpredictable way and could end up farther back than when it started!

The amoeba

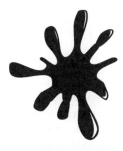

To refer to an organisation as an amoeba may not seem terribly complimentary, however, this model does contain many of the advantageous qualities. The initial difference from the cube and ball is the amoeba's ability to move without relying upon external forces: it has an innate energy. The nucleus is constantly changing position and when faced with an obstacle it does one of two things: it either absorbs it or goes around it. The organism is flexible, with methods to protect itself and to evaluate things in its path before proceeding to embrace or avoid them.

We know that some practices seem to thrive on change and challenge, whilst others buckle under and fail to respond positively. Looking at the organisational models it is clear that balanced flexibility is the key. Being too reactive can be just as catastrophic as being too rigid. Comparing a practice to the models will give an indication of how the team will respond to conflict, but first we should look at the common causes. This section will review how partners interact, not take a wider view of the whole practice team.

CAUSES OF PARTNERSHIP CONFLICT

It should be stated at the outset that all the issues described below only become important to individuals when they feel that they are being disadvantaged. A genuinely happy partnership, defined as one with no negative conflict at all, only occurs when each partner feels valued and works within a tolerant 'give and take' system. The reader may wish to refer to the 'symptoms of conflict' in Chapter 2, where the behavioural indicators of conflict are described. If a given partnership is exhibiting several such signs it may be time to pinpoint the root causes. As in all problem-solving exercises it is logical to start with the most likely cause and end with the least likely. For this reason the workload, finance and future direction of the practice are given pride of place.

Workload

Not all general practitioners work full-time solely on providing general medical services to their personal list of patients; if they did there would be few disparities. Once the list sizes were deemed to be equal, so would the workload be. This, of course, is not the case. Partnerships are a combination of full- and part-time partners, outside commitments, GMS and non-GMS income and varying levels of responsibility towards the business aspects of the practice. Comparisons become difficult and each partner's perception of their own contribution is distorted by their personal bias.

Example:

Dr A does a clinical assistantship in ophthalmology at the local hospital for two half-days each week and generates approximately £6500 per annum. Dr B does one extra surgery each week from 5.30 pm to 7.30 pm as part of general medical services to respond to the needs of a commuting population.

Dr A feels that the additional income and his improved clinical skills are an advantage to the practice. Dr B sees his partner having two easy afternoons pursuing his own interests whilst he is having to work an extra evening to cope with routine patient demands, because the net loss to the practice has been two surgeries every week, which would have offered 30 appointments.

Dr B feels that Dr A is making a fuss about nothing. He brings a substantial amount of money into the practice without the need to employ a locum. Dr A chose to do an evening surgery which Dr B thinks must be the ideal way to practice medicine – no telephone interruptions, extras to see or emergency visits.

Here we begin to see some of the emotional reactions to complicated situations and these will also depend upon the individual's financial needs. A partner who needs to earn more will almost certainly be willing to contribute more, whereas a partner who is financially secure may place a higher value on leisure time.

The 1990 New GP Contract forced all partnerships to review their working methods by cutting almost 50 per cent from basic allowances and offering payment for new items of service, targets and postgraduate education allowances to recoup the loss. The number of patients registered has the greatest impact on workload and finance. This is a fundamental decision that has to be taken collectively as it affects just about everything else in the practice, from the doctor time required to the practice premises. A growing list size may require more physical space, additional telephone lines and more practice nurses. A falling list size could mean the non-replacement of the next partner to resign or retire, staff redundancies or renting out spare space to other health professionals. All of these are fundamental to the strategic planning of resources. Matching list size to doctor time is not a static equation that can be calculated on a national formula, it will vary from season to season and reflect the practice profile.

Examples:

An East coast practice has a list size of 22,000 patients and sees 15,000 temporary residents between Easter and the end of August every year.

One university town practice has a list size that halves between June and October when the students return home for the summer vacation.

A seaside practice on the South coast has higher than average numbers of elderly as the area is a popular retirement haven. The workload increases considerably, especially for the practice nurse team, when it is time to vaccinate the at-risk patients against influenza.

Another fundamental decision that goes hand in hand with the list size is the way that patients will be registered and by whom they will be seen. If a practice operates a strict personal list system the number of patients registered with each doctor needs to be equal or in direct proportion to their commitment. Within that total some alignment of the elderly and under fives should be considered as these are the 'labour intensive' groups.

Example:

To iron out the imbalances between personal lists one practice manager decided to meet every new patient wishing to join the practice and, according to their ages, guided them towards a particular doctor. This stopped any imbalances from growing, e.g. the doctor with the highest number of over 65s was not given any additional patients over 55, and over a period of five years the lists (and workload) were more evenly matched.

The partnerships who operate a 'preferred doctor' or completely open system may find balancing workload much easier. The booking of appointments is centralised and the routine appointments for all doctors are filled before 'extras' are allocated, again on a strict rota basis. Routine clinics, like child development and minor operations, are delegated to one partner on behalf of the practice to gain the economies of scale and to make the most effective use of resources and special interests. This does not address the issue of outside commitments and their impact on the distribution of surgery slots and home visits, but goes some way to bring these issues into the open, and a visible system can reassure. In other words, any partner who feels that he or she is doing more than someone else can go to the centralised appointment desk and check for themselves. This does not apply to strict personal-list systems where the ability to balance workload is limited, and the potential for one partner to do far more, or far less, is greater.

Certain geographic areas are deemed to have special problems and can claim additional income in the form of deprivation payments, so the degree of difficulty is well recognised. The exact nature of the increased demands can be hard to quantify because it is manifested in any number of small ways that, combined together, have a major impact.

Example:

One GP who works in a practice with a large section of the population living in a designated area of deprivation made these comments. He felt that the patients had an attitude towards the general practitioner that was almost impossible to alter, even after 10 years of trying to educate them. The patients brought a great many social issues to their doctors because they were more accessible than the other welfare services and were perceived to have unlimited powers. When the patients came to the GP they wanted a 'quick fix' and only a minority complied with a longer-term plan to improve their overall standard of health. The number of out-of-hours calls was higher than average as hardly any of the patients paid for prescriptions and they would call out the doctor if they needed medication, e.g. Calpol for a poorly child, not because they did not know what to do but because they would get a free prescription or a sample from the doctor's bag.

The social, financial and housing problems of the patients are closely related to their general well-being and inevitably find their way into the consultation as they are contributory factors that cannot be ignored.

The numbers of part-time partners and the introduction of job-sharing have some unique characteristics in terms of workload. These posts cannot be viewed as options taken only by women, as many men choose a reduced partnership commitment for many of the same reasons as their female colleagues. Technically a part-time partner is contracted to work for a stipulated number of weekly hours, and usually they are expected to take a pro-rata share of management responsibilities, out-of-hours duties, home visits, 'extra' consultations and paperwork. The majority of part-time partners would claim that they always exceed their contracted hours and do 'more than their fair share'. Some consider the imbalance a small price to pay, others want the imbalance corrected or financial arrangements altered. There is no doubt that the pressure on a part-time partner to tie up all the loose ends before handing over to someone else or leaving for the day is greater than that on a full-time partner who can take advantage of quieter times during the week to catch up. Part-time partners are only needed for additional cover on busy days or times, so they are unlikely to have equitable quiet spells.

Example

The practice is particularly busy and all of the partners, four full-time and two part-time, are working hard. The numbers of patients seen as 'extras' are increasing and all of the consultations have been appropriate.

Dr A is full-time and usually sees her last patient at 6.00 pm, which means that she leaves to go home after tidying up her paperwork at around 6.30 pm For the past two weeks she has not finished consulting until 7.15 pm and leaves the building at about 7.45 pm.

Dr B is part-time and works five mornings until 1.00 pm. He has to leave at this time to get to his afternoon commitments, which are a clinical assistantship post and sessions as a medical examiner for an insurance company. He too sees a number of extras but leaves at 1.00 pm, if necessary, leaving paperwork until the next morning. The increased consultations have reduced the amount of time Dr B has available to do home visits, and on three days these have been distributed among the other partners.

Dr A is annoyed about the unfairness of the situation. She has to work late if the patient demand requires her to do so, but she will not get any compensating time off or an increase in drawings. She feels that Dr B is protected by his part-time commitment and should do proportionately more before he leaves each day.

Dr B knows that the practice is busy and feels that he takes a fair share of the extra work. His partners know that he has to leave at 1.00 pm and he refuses to stay later than this unless he is given additional time off or an increase in drawings.

Some practices appoint a part-time partner to increase their flexibility and may stipulate some regular sessions every week and use one or two 'floating' sessions that can be used to cover holidays and potential pressure points. To others this concept is too cumbersome administratively or they are unable to find a partner who could accommodate this degree of variety.

When outside commitments are evaluated in terms of workload and cost-effectiveness every partner will hold a different view. The doctors who are completely fulfilled by the general practitioner role may find it hard to understand why colleagues need the challenge of another area of medicine. In the commercial world it is considered vital for senior personnel to either change jobs within a company or move companies on a regular basis. This is an accepted process to avoid becoming stale and to continuously enhance and develop skills. Indeed, no one in industry can rely on long-term employment stability and/or expect to spend their entire working life in one environment. The only method open to a general practitioner to emulate this constant learning process is to take on responsibilities outside the practice. They may be in direct line with the provision of general medical services, e.g. becoming medical officer to a private nursing home for the elderly or locality commissioning. There are opportunities to move into education by becoming a GP trainer or Course Organiser, or into the medico-political arena via the Local Medical Council. It is the way that these outside commitments are negotiated or subsequently reviewed within the partnership that causes conflict. Too often the individual presents a biased perspective to colleagues, playing on the potential benefits and ignoring the disadvantages. The discussions become subjective, and if the partner is well respected agreement is likely to be forthcoming. The attitude may be different if a new or less highly regarded partner puts forward the same proposal. The lack of a fair system to evaluate any outside commitment will always leave partnerships vulnerable to discreet unfairness, and the collective decision will be influenced by the offence and perceived rejection by the peer group that a refusal may cause. The partners who express a wish to take on a new responsibility, but are willing to accept their partners' refusal with good grace if it cannot be accommodated, are more likely to be refused. The partners who present a strong case and who make it very clear that this is what they wish to do are more likely to gain agreement.

Outside commitments are contagious. Partners without an additional interest that takes them away from the practice may resent their colleagues who do have one; the natural reaction is to seek to do the same. There are immense benefits to any partnership if the insights and new skills can be shared and the additional income is direct profit. In real terms it may reduce a partnership to a team of part-time principals. This will affect flexibility, communication, the level of locum cover, times and days of regular meetings and their accessibility to patients. If these issues are properly discussed before a partner accepts an outside commitment proper plans can be made and conflict minimised. If they are not, resentment will build and surface at a later date. To then insist that a partner relinquish a particular duty will be much more demoralising to all concerned.

Some practices can inflate their workload by being too available. Whilst it may seem the ideal to see the majority of patients on the same day as they request an appointment, it may encourage the patients to seek the doctor's advice before trying any self-help measures. The patients will feel that their doctors provide an excellent service, but they may also receive the wrong message about consulting a doctor appropriately. Eventually the workload will fall back again if doctors deal with the immediate problem presented to them, and then invest time to explain what to do should a similar situation arise in the future. Longer term the patients will be educated about minor illness. If the partners are constantly seeing self-limiting problems and referring patients back to a chemist for over-the-counter remedies, the work itself will become frustrating and take time that could be used to develop new services.

As in all problem-solving activity the only way to initiate discussion about workloads is to begin with some accurate data collection. Every GP computer software package will produce detailed age/sex breakdowns, which is a good place to start. If each partner runs on a strict personal list system, i.e. the patient sees the doctor with whom they are registered, the analysis will highlight anomalies. Irrespective of the way that an appointments system is run, manual or computerised, it is possible to record the number of sessions that the doctor was available and the number of patients seen in surgeries, home visits, extras and clinics. These statistics can be logged daily or weekly by the receptionists on a standardised form produced in-house (Box 5.1).

There are any number of methods for trying to rationalise workload and patient demands and this type of form can assist a practice wishing to audit the impact of new systems. For example, if a practice offered a specific time for telephone consultations or pre-screening

Box 5.1

Week commencing Monday					
	Number of patients seen:				
	Booked appointments	Extras	Clinics	Home Visits	Emergency Visits
MONDAY					
TUESDAY					
WEDNESDAY					
THURSDAY					
FRIDAY					
SATURDAY					
Totals:					

by a suitably qualified practice nurse, these innovations could be added to the data-collection sheet to build a 'before' and 'after' picture. It would quantify the impact and facilitate an evidence-based decision.

Finance

Workload and finance are interrelated, not just by the fundamental baseline, which is the number of patients, but by the effectiveness of the whole team of partners to maximise item of service income opportunistically. The average list size within the United Kingdom varies from 1524 in Scotland to 1887 in England. Yet without an appropriate number of patients the potential for income generation is limited. The age breakdown will affect the workload. For example, in a retirement area the higher rates of capitation payments for the elderly will compensate for lower than average maternity or contraceptive income.

The biggest practice investment will be the premises, assuming that they are owned by the partnership. The cost rent and notional rent schemes allow partners to seek funding to purchase or extend premises, and provide a monthly payment. As with all such subsidies there are criteria that must be met and it is likely that any partnership planning to build premises will have to find some additional capital in the form of a mortgage or personal loan. This implies that the ownership of premises is borne equally between partners, which is not always the case. Historically one or more partners may own the premises and take a larger proportion, or all, of the health authority payments for rent. When a partner joins a practice they may have to 'buy in' the outgoing partner's share; others may join a partnership which has a self-funding pension scheme so that this is not necessary. Whatever the arrangements they must be properly vetted and overseen by the practice accountant to ensure that any system is completely fair to all partners.

This brings us to the philosophy that applies to each partnership's financial affairs. The majority work on a totally pooled arrangement, some retain their personal payments for seniority or postgraduate education allowance, some work a system where each partner retains their own item of service payments. It really does not matter, as long as the methods apply equally to all partners and the various calculations are available for scrutiny. The conflict arises when this does not happen.

Example:

In a three-partner practice, Dr D, the senior partner, had always been responsible for the finance. He was originally single-handed and worked without a practice manager. As the practice had grown two other partners and a practice manager were appointed, but the senior partner continued to keep all ledgers, pay staff and had all of the bank statements sent to his home address. The newest partner, Dr E, had asked repeatedly for sight of the partnership accounts, but they had not been forthcoming after two years. His motivation was his own level of drawings, which was well below the published intended figure, when his senior partner was living a lavish lifestyle. There was a very acrimonious partnership meeting when Dr D became defensive and asked his partners if they did not trust him. Dr E responded that if everything was above board, what was the problem?

Sadly this partnership was dissolved when the two newer partners resigned. Dr D reverted to a single-handed status.

The simplest way to manage partnership finance is a totally pooled arrangement, where every bit of income generated by the partners on approved medically-related activities, irrespective of the source or reason, is paid into the partnership account. All profits, and the occasional surpluses that build up in the accounts, are distributed in partnership percentage ratios. This also guarantees that each partner has the correct amount of superannuation attributed to their NHS pension. A totally pooled situation ensures that decisions are made collectively about workload issues, like outside commitments, because everyone has a stake in the outcome.

Income for general medical services is clearly defined and the intended remuneration is a figure which is published annually, gross and net. In order to maximise income the manager needs to understand the Statement of Fees and Allowances (commonly called The Red Book) and to train the staff accordingly. All such income must be monitored in-year, as it is too late to take any corrective actions if this happens only when the practice accounts are audited. The NHS income statements arrive at the end of each quarter and the capitation statements arrive at the beginning of each quarter; both need to be verified speedily as queries must be raised within fourteen days. Some managers transfer the information to a computerised spreadsheet which gradually builds a picture of seasonal trends and comparisons between partner's lists. Health Authority errors will be obvious and easily queried. The advantage of such a system will be the historical data and the ability to evaluate the effects of new administrative systems or the effect of a new partner. This in turn facilitates effective planning for income and cash flow. It may also highlight staff training needs, for example, if a new receptionist takes over the responsibility for maternity claims but the income drops dramatically despite a constant number of pregnant patients, the chances are that the administration is at fault.

Recently we have seen guidance on 'core' and 'non-core' activities. There has been a growing concern that general practice will bear the brunt of the shift in workload from secondary to primary care, without additional funding or resources. This has allowed GPs to question all of the non-core work and seek appropriate remuneration. Very briefly, core services are defined under five main headings and encompass the essential primary care that every patient can expect:

- Services normally provided by every GP when responding to a problem presented by, or on behalf of, one of their patients;
- Proactive services which are normally provided by every GP, e.g. new patient checks and health promotion advice;
- Services which are normally provided by every practice but not necessarily by each GP in the practice, e.g. maternity services, contraception, minor operations;
- Organising patient services as provided for in the Red Book or NHS regulations, e.g. out-of-hours care, organising cervical cytology;
- Organising the work of staff employed by the practice.

All other work is deemed to be 'non-core' and includes things like drug trials and research or work which requires specialist training. These should be the subject of an explicit contract with a Health Authority or other purchaser. For some practices this may result in additional income or offer some avenues to pursue any entrepreneurial ambitions. The manager has a key role in becoming fully conversant with the guidelines and prompting negotiations for non-core services already being undertaken or identifying potential new sources of income.

In order to remain viable every general practitioner needs to maintain a comprehensive working knowledge of finance. The thought of a GP thinking and behaving like a business person was, at one time, distasteful. In recent years it has become imperative and is reflected in the vocational training syllabus. If the practice manager is not financially aware the partners may need to delegate one of their own group to oversee the financial aspects of their practice. There are a number of sources of advice and guidance, namely the practice accountant, independent financial adviser, Health Authority or bank manager.

Future direction of the practice

The partners must work as a team for all the same reasons that the staff need to work together. The start of this process is in the identification of shared and longer-term aims. Yet, surprisingly, this type of discussion does not happen routinely in all partnerships. The short-term aims are reviewed annually to meet the needs of the business plan which is submitted to the Health Authority at the end of each year. This, however, does not challenge partners to examine and openly discuss their personal agendas and aspirations. For this reason, when a major initiative or imposed directive enters the general practice arena the reactions can be extreme. There is an element of bemusement when a colleague's opinion does not match one's own, this can develop into anger or resentment if it is treated too lightly or ignored.

Failure to address fundamental differences of opinion will almost certainly result in resignation, voluntary early retirement or a partnership split. The larger partnerships are more vulnerable than small ones, possibly because the direct communication is not as frequent or the personal rapport is not strong enough for real cohesion. The simple logistics of planning meetings when all partners are available will be difficult in a large partnership, as spreading holiday entitlement and study leave evenly throughout the year will result in someone being away at almost any time.

Poor performance

As we have seen in Chapter 2, poor performance is a symptom of conflict, but how do partnerships respond? If a member of staff needs disciplining or re-training it will be dealt with by the manager, but who deals with a poorly performing partner?

The ability of any partner to disclose their own feelings of inadequacy or lack of confidence will depend upon their trust in and respect for their peer group. Some practices are extremely good at analysing personal performance by using educational and feedback forums. This may take the form of case reviews, examining the reasons for sudden deaths or clinical audit. Regular exposure to sharing and seeking ideas on the management of complicated diagnoses will help to avoid mistakes and instances of poor judgment recurring. Within a group practice there will be a range of expertise available as each partner tends to have a special medical interest. If an atmosphere can be created that encourages a frank exchange of views the poorly performing partner will feel more supported than criticised.

Another common reason for a doctor's interest waning is a lack of stimulation. After a period of years undertaking the same range of services for the same group of patients boredom can set in. Initiatives like computerisation and fundholding or commissioning have given partners the opportunity to gain a different insight or perspective on their traditional role. Those who enjoy audit have the Internet and access to computerised databases to assist the development of their skills. It is possible that a group of partners who are locked in to their own general practice and who shun outside commitments or voluntary responsibilities become stale together. A career as a general practitioner can be a daunting prospect, especially for a recently vocationally trained doctor who has become used to changing departments and work groups on a six-monthly rotation. This group see change as a positive learning experience and are likely to want to continue this pattern, not necessarily by changing working environment but certainly by having opportunities at regular intervals to seek new challenges.

It is unrealistic to expect any person to openly state their own shortcomings; if these manifests themselves in unsatisfactory performance or behaviour then it will take a colleague to initiate the dialogue. Almost the only time that a senior partner is perceived to have special powers is when a more junior partner is causing problems. The other partners tend towards upward delegation and suggest that it is the senior partner's place to 'speak quietly to them'. This assumes that the delegated partner has all the right qualities to solve the problem tactfully and honestly, and without any personal bias.

Example:

Sally has been a partner for eight years, working on a half-time basis. Over the last six months the staff have noticed that she is behind with her administration, especially referral letters and medical attendant's reports. When she was on holiday there were a number of patients who grumbled that they had not received their expected appointments with consultants, and a number of insurance companies telephoned to chase up overdue medical reports. The other partners ended up dealing with the urgent items and realised the scale of the Sally's backlog. At the practice meeting that was routinely held in her absence Sally's partners agreed that something had to be done as she was not pulling her weight. The senior partner, Richard, was delegated to talk to Sally on her return from holiday.

Richard thought that his colleagues were making a fuss about nothing, and shared his view with Sally. He cited one person as the prime mover in wanting her to sharpen up her act and quoted this person as saying that she was clearly getting away with doing less than everyone else. He made no attempt to discuss her total workload or ask why she had allowed her admin to slip.

Sally was furious and refused to speak to the partner who was supposed to be causing trouble.

No one enjoys criticising a colleague and too often partnerships ignore a problem in the hope that it will disappear; of course, it usually gets worse. The assumption that the senior partner is the best person to take control of the situation is also a dangerous one. Even if he or she is, no sensitive discussion should be undertaken by just one person. A third person who enjoys the respect of the partner being criticised will provide a balance to what is said, and will go some way to preventing personal interpretation overtaking the partnership wishes. What happens if the senior partner's performance is causing concern? The prospect of dealing with it can be so daunting that it never gets tackled and the remaining partners start displaying some of the symptoms of conflict, like the formation of cliques and backbiting. In extreme cases the adverse, sometimes spiteful, comments are inappropriately made to the general staff.

Basic employment and team disciplines are difficult to apply to partners. For example, how can a 'boss' be asked to improve their timekeeping? It is, after all, their business. A manager seeking support to tackle the issue may not find it from the other partners, partly because they may not suffer from the ramifications of angry patients and partly because they may not see their colleague arriving late. Yet, the manager will know that the errant partner will rapidly gain a reputation for being late and running late, the patients will gauge the amount of time that they are likely to be kept waiting and start arriving late for their booked appointments. Ultimately, the public perception of the efficiency of the practice will be damaged.

Example:

Dr B wanted a Friday morning off, but this was not agreed by his partners because it would have left only one partner available to patients. He was still determined to take the time off and asked several friends and family to telephone and make an appointment for that morning. He explained that he did not want them to appear, just to book an appointment. The previous day he checked the surgery list and noticed one or two legitimate patients; these he visited at home and told them not to cancel their appointment as he would do it. Dr B arrived on time on the Friday morning, told the reception team that he would not accept any telephone calls during his surgery, took his box of medical records into his consulting room and promptly walked out of the back door.

The morning was exceptionally busy, the manager was on holiday and when the staff were looking for Dr B at the end of surgery they assumed that he had gone out on his routine home visits. In short, no one realised that anything was amiss. His ruse was only successful because patients did not have to check in at the reception desk; traditionally they simply sat in the waiting room until they were called by the doctor.

This deception worked so well that Dr B decided to repeat it the next time he wanted time off that was inconvenient to the practice. This time the practice manager was in the building and realised that the waiting room was too quiet and decided to investigate. She checked his list of appointments and began to understand what was happening.

On the third occasion that Dr B booked a spoof surgery the manager was waiting at the back door to intercept him as he left.

At the next partnership meeting it was agreed that in future all patients would check in at the reception desk.

Appraisal for general staff is now an accepted way of improving and maintaining standards, yet it is not common for partners to initiate appraisal of their own performance. If it were, poor performance would not be tolerated or allowed to drag on without intervention. The least threatening way to introduce appraisal for partners would be self-appraisal. The partnership could agree the priority areas for review and each partner would assess themselves and then have an opportunity to match their own perceptions against those of their colleagues. It may be appropriate for the manager to be included, or it may not. From the self-assessment would come a personal learning plan and a set of short-term and long-term objectives which could be discussed annually. The benefit of introducing appraisal is that it is a natural extension of business planning and gives the partnership team a sense of purpose and direction. Communication automatically improves, constructive criticism becomes normal, management issues can be incorporated and each individual can take time to evaluate their own professional aspirations.

Poor physical or mental health

If a partner is becoming ill it may not be the individual who realises first; it is more likely to be noticed by other members of the team. In fact, the manager and general staff will have greater opportunities to observe a partner's behaviour and demeanour. There is a natural reluctance to ask a physician about their health because non-clinicians often feel slightly silly suggesting 'lots of fluid and a couple of paracetamol', for example. However common self-limiting physical illnesses, like a cold or chest infection, are easy to see and understand and even major problems, like a hip replacement or hysterectomy, can be discussed openly as they have a definite cause and solution and no stigma is attached. Colleagues are usually sympathetic and willing to alter their working patterns to cover a defined period of time. This is not always so when a partner suffers from a stress-related or mental illness. Part of the problem is the gradual onset of symptoms, the attitude of, 'If I can cope, why can't they?' and the lack of opportunity to observe partnership colleagues. If sick leave is taken it is often open-ended, and goodwill between partners is soon exhausted if workload increases with the prospect of more of the same to come. There are many clues that can alert a team to the fact that one of their number is not coping (Box 5.2).

Box 5.2

Physical signs	Mental signs
Breathlessness	*Indecision*
Palpitations	*Loss of concentration*
Nausea	*Tunnel vision*
Muscle twitches	*Bad dreams*
Sweating	*Worry*
Vague aches and pains	*Muddled thinking*
Headaches	*Loss of memory*
Frequent infections	
Emotional signs	**Behavioural signs**
Irritability	*Unsociability*
Gloom	*Restlessness*
Tension	*Change in eating habits*
Loss of enthusiasm	*Reliance on stimulants*
Loss of confidence	*Loss of libido*
Reduced self-esteem	*Sleep disturbance*
Alienation	*Lying*
	Accident prone

One of the problems of stress is that the individual affected becomes less aware of these changes in themselves and less adept at pinpointing the causes. The first step in helping a stressed colleague is to get them to communicate their fears and feelings, but this cannot happen if there are no appropriate opportunities or if their colleagues lack empathy. For example, an hour's lunch-time meeting is not the forum in which to encourage a partner to talk openly and honestly about their innermost feelings. An evening meeting that has no definite finish would be better, as there will be time to discuss coping mechanisms in depth. Alternatively, a stressed partner can be directed to a professional source of advice or treatment. There may be a practice counsellor or, if this is too local, a national support organisation specifically for members of the medical profession.

It is considered a rare compliment if a GP is approached by a medical colleague and asked to care for them and their families. New partners are occasionally encouraged to register with another partner in the same practice. This works well until that partner needs impartial advice. The dilemma of treating a colleague professionally, especially when the information gained during a consultation has an adverse impact on the partnership, is an unfair burden. The only situation that is more worrying is the doctor who does not register at all with another GP and self-diagnoses and self-treats. In order to protect doctors' health they should be registered with a doctor away from their own practice.

Unsafe clinical practice

Given the advent of vocational training and the recent introduction of summative assessment, it is increasingly unlikely that an unsafe clinician will be appointed as a partner. The most accurate barometer of any partner's clinical performance is the number and nature of patient complaints. The NHS complaints procedure has insisted that patient dissatisfactions are dealt with promptly and discussed by the team.

Doctors are only human and certainly not infallible. There are errors of judgment and, with the benefit of hindsight, a wish that things had been done differently. If there are regular case reviews and opportunities for partners to seek the opinion of their peers the mistakes can become a learning tool for all.

Conflict within partnerships may arise when a colleague's competence is questioned. If this is substantiated by a patient complaint it can be dealt with openly and in the ways agreed by the practice. As we know, not all patients with a justified grievance complain. Instead, another partner or the manager may be aware of an instance that causes concern and not have a clearly defined method of dealing with it. Experienced staff may also alert someone in authority if they know that a clinician is not following recommended codes of practice.

Example:

Dr Y was overheard giving the newly appointed partner advice on how to cope with out-of-hours calls, especially ones in the early hours of the morning. 'Just call an ambulance if it sounds serious, or tell the patient to 'phone when the surgery opens and insist that they are fitted in as an emergency if it sounds minor. This will mean that you never have to get out of bed.'

The partner who accidentally heard what was said decided to raise the issue at the next practice meeting under the guise of an audit of out-of-hours home visits and the income that they generated. The opportunity was used to emphasise the GP's responsibilities towards a patient who felt that they needed emergency medical attention.

Some doubts are more imagined than real. These may be a consequence of a natural dislike for a colleague or a wish to score points. There is no substitute for facts and evidence when criticising anyone, and information must be verified before any action is taken.

Example:

Peter was growing increasingly annoyed at the performance of one of his colleagues, Neil. He privately felt that Neil was not thorough enough when making a diagnosis and that it was only a matter of time until it resulted in a claim of medical negligence. Peter had never discussed this openly, mainly because there was no evidence at all to substantiate his fears.

One day, when Peter was particularly busy, he told the practice secretary, 'Neil's retirement can't come soon enough, he's a walking liability'. This was passed quickly to every other member of staff and resulted in divided loyalties. The practice manager went to Peter and suggested that he address his comments directly to Neil and that he should apologise to the secretary for speaking out of turn. He did neither, he ignored Neil and the relationships across the whole practice became very strained.

More usual are breaches of the Terms of Service, which is the contract a general practitioner enters into with the NHS when he or she is approved as a partner (Box 5.3).

Box 5.3

NHS patients should be able to expect the following:
- to be registered with a doctor of their choice, within certain guidelines;
- to change doctors without giving a reason;
- to be offered a new patient health check within 4 weeks of joining a doctor's list;
- the elderly (aged 75 years and over) should be invited annually for a health check or offered a home visit;
- medical cover 24 hours a day, 7 days a week, either by their own doctor or a designated deputy;
- adequate medical records must be maintained and returned promptly when recalled by the health authority;
- to be prescribed appropriate drugs and medicines;
- to be referred to a consultant or specialist if it is deemed appropriate by the GP;
- to be given, or have access to, a leaflet explaining all the patient services available at the practice;
- to be seen by the community nursing team in their own home where there are special needs, e.g. MS.

All staff need to be aware of a doctor's obligations to his or her patients and the systems in the practice must support them. This is an essential part of initial training for all staff as they can assist the partners in the fulfillment of their Terms of Service. This encompasses passing on messages accurately and dealing with patient requests for urgent medical treatment promptly.

THE PARTNERSHIP AGREEMENT

When there are partnership conflicts the first port of call for guidance is the partnership agreement. Every practice should have such a document that is updated and signed whenever there is a partnership change. Not to have an agreement makes all of the partners vulnerable as there will be no set policy for holidays, study leave, financial matters, resignations and arbitration, among many others. It is the foundation for defining standards and to ensure fairness to all partners, irrespective of their length of service, and it is the equivalent of a contract of employment for the staff.

There are many occasions when reference to a partnership agreement can solve partnership conflict. An example would be a partner wishing to query their steps to parity; there should be clear guidance about the percentage increases in partnership drawings and at what point they become effective.

It would be impossible to draft a generic partnership agreement because every single practice is affected by a unique set of circumstances that must be reflected in the document. It is a formalisation of what actually happens combined with contingency plans to deal with foreseeable events and essential clauses to ensure equity for all parties. Any practice should seek advice when drawing up a partnership agreement, ideally from a solicitor who is particularly skilled in partnership law and medical practices. The BMA also provide guidance for their members, as do the various medical defence organisations.

There are some clauses that can be considered essential:

- date of document;
- name and title of the organisation;
- practice address;
- nature of the business;
- commencement and duration of agreement;
- practice capital;
- premises;
- income and expenses;

- division of receipts;
- attention to the affairs of the organisation;
- taxation;
- employing and dismissing staff;
- power to make decisions;
- holidays, study leave and sabbaticals;
- incapacity;
- maternity leave;
- leaving the partnership
  - voluntarily
  - involuntarily;
- retirement on age grounds;
- restrictive covenants;
- defence societies;
- arbitration;
- banking;
- accounts;
- superannuation.

Legal advice is essential when drafting or reviewing a partnership agreement; the same is also true in the event of a dispute that results in a partnership split or dissolution.

Dissolving a partnership

A partnership agreement will cover the breakdown in commitment to working in association with other medical practitioners and set out the terms to apportion assets. There will be guidance on dealing with a partner who resigns or retires on the wishes of the other partners. These circumstances may be distressing to all concerned but there will be provision for the partnership to continue and disruption to the patients and staff will be minimised.

There may also be restrictive covenants which will apply to a resigning partner. These usually relate to a specific period of time and radius from the existing practice premises when and where an outgoing partner cannot accept a partnership patient onto their NHS list, assuming that they continue their career as a GP. Any such restriction has to be enforceable if it is to be meaningful, and the accepted recommendation is a period of two years following resignation and a radius of two miles.

If a serious conflict occurs that cannot be resolved to the satisfaction of all partners, then a partnership split or dissolution may be the best course of action. Such events cannot be assumed to be totally negative, indeed, it may be the right decision if various factions have polarised and wish to progress in entirely different directions. However, the step often missed is to enforce the arbitration clause in the partnership agreement. This offers mediation by an independent person and the practice solicitor should be able to provide details.

If a partnership splits but remains in the same premises, for convenience or because of financial commitment, there should be an agreement explicitly stating the terms and conditions.

Example:

Dr A and Dr B were in partnership together and had jointly purchased new premises. When they argued and decided to work as independent single-handed practitioners they realised that neither could afford to move out and find new premises, hence they must continue in the same building.

A brick wall was erected down the middle of the building.

Example:

A eight-partner practice split into two groups of four. The premises were purpose-built and represented the main asset of a pension fund to which they all belonged. The two new partnerships agreed to continue in the same premises and take advantage of the economies of scale by jointly employing certain staff, like the computer manager.

Apart from the lists of partners by the front door, re-arranged into two partnerships, and two practice brochures instead of one, the patients remained largely unaware of the divide.

If partners have never signed a partnership agreement the partnership is deemed to be a 'partnership at will'. This means that any partner can dissolve the partnership at any time, with immediate effect. The practical implications of such a move are dramatic as the premises and all of the assets must be sold to settle the liabilities. Under the Partnership Act 1980 the sale should be by auction and any bidding by the partners is restricted. This may mean that the partners have nowhere to practice. It is possible that, after a dissolution and until the premises are sold, each principle runs an independent practice in the same building if they cannot afford to purchase or rent anywhere else.

New partners

There are some aspects of conflict and partnership agreements that apply specifically to new partners. It is usual to discuss terms and conditions, e.g. holiday entitlement and steps to parity, during the selection process. If the partnership has an agreement these are simple to answer and will apply equally to all partners. The candidate can then make an informed decision about joining the practice. It is entirely reasonable for a prospective new partner to ask for a copy of the partnership agreement to read thoroughly before accepting any offer and to seek an independent legal or professional opinion. For a partnership to be unable to comply with such a request should raise doubts in the prospective partner's mind. The same is true of practice accounts.

If prospective partners query clauses within the agreement or an accounting mechanism and the response is, 'We can look at that when you've joined us,' they would be unwise to assume that it will be reviewed to their satisfaction or at all.

Example:

Angela accepted a partnership post on a promise that the maternity arrangements, which were extremely punitive, would be changed. At the end of six months the other partners refused to alter the partnership agreement, based on their previous experience of a partner who had taken maternity leave and treated the practice badly.

Angela resigned because she was planning to have a family in the future and could foresee that she would be financially out of pocket if she took maternity leave.

The tone and content of any partnership agreement will disclose the attitudes and beliefs of existing partners.

To take a partnership post straight after vocational training and after a relatively short recruitment process is daunting. The candidate may not have a clear idea about the type of practice that will suit them and the existing partners may not be skilled at selection. This is recognised by a mutual assessment period, usually of six months. This gives all the partners time to judge one another in more depth before the partnership position is confirmed, agreements signed and financial investments made. The last point applies to the new partner purchasing property in the area as well as a potential financial contribution to the practice.

GPs tend to feel very confident in their abilities to assess partnership candidates because there are shared experiences that can be explored and compared. Even so, some of the most pertinent questions are never asked, for example:

> Has a patient ever complained about you?
> Have you ever been involved in a clash of personalities?
> How have you resolved a difficult situation?
> What do you consider to be the important qualities in a team member?

All of these would identify certain characteristics and personal behaviour, which may or may not be desirable. It is fair to assume that any minor irritating habits that surface at an interview can turn into major annoyances if that person is appointed. The theory of interviewing is to make a decision based upon evidence, but general practice is such a close-knit environment at every level that instinct is just as important. The bottom-line question will always be, 'Can I trust, respect and enjoy working with that person for the foreseeable future?'

In the past, when the wife or husband of a GP was expected to take out-of-hour telephone calls, it was considered necessary to include them in the selection process. This is often referred to as 'trial by sherry'. The relevance is diminishing for a variety of reasons: co-operatives have removed the need for GPs to have someone to intercept their calls, and there are a greater number of female doctors and an increasing number of working wives. This has the effect of encouraging partnerships to appoint a new partner on their merits, not because they have a socially acceptable partner.

References can provide valuable information if the correct questions are asked. A glowing and vague verbal reference may be reassuring but it does not have the comprehensive quality that a list of specific questions would provoke. In a busy practice with relatively large patient lists, questions about the candidate's physical stamina, ability to prioritise and cope with pressure would be relevant; in a practice with a large elderly population, questions about their experience of geriatric medicine; in a new town with lots of first-time buyers, questions about ante-natal and post-natal care and rapport with the under fives. To gain a cross-section of views at least three references need to be taken including those from both secondary and primary care. The other network that may be helpful to tap into is the practice manager's. It will use non-clinical criteria and place more emphasis on communication and team skills.

Choices are not always well made and new partners do not always meet expectations. A new partner, especially in their first partnership post, will need assistance and to be shown some tolerance while they become acclimatised. There are some measures that will hasten a sense of belonging:

Induction period:
To allow the new partner to spend the first few days meeting all the practice and community staff, finding out the consultants and hospitals for referrals, training on the practice computer software, reviewing copies of protocols, and a map of the area, meeting the accountant, solicitor and bank manager, etc.

Mentor:
To appoint another partner as a mentor will offer a new partner a source of information and reassurance. It provides a method of asking 'silly' and obvious questions privately. The mentor can gently guide and advise, and ensure that the new partner is given every opportunity to do well.

Interim assessment:
This can take the format of a discussion at a practice meeting after the new partner has been with the practice for two or three months. They need to be given advance warning and time to prepare any issues they wish to raise with colleagues. If the other partners have concerns or criticisms this may be better handled by a smaller meeting involving two or three partners.

If, despite all of these techniques, the new partner is not proving to be satisfactory it must be tackled quickly. Examples of poor performance or behaviour must be gathered and clear aims for improvement given. These should be linked to a period of time when a further assessment will be made. There may be some legitimate reasons why the new partner is experiencing difficulty and these should be listened to and acted upon, if appropriate. A new partner moving into an unfamiliar part of the country may take longer to settle than someone local. They may be living apart from their families and not have a network of colleagues to access, and they will know nothing about local consultants and services. Any judgment must be balanced and take every contributory factor into account.

If the only option is for the new partner to leave the practice then it should be done with dignity and consideration. The staff and patients will want to know the reasons and the partners must agree a public statement that everyone will adhere to. The practice will have a code of confidentiality and this is simply another aspect of it.

The outgoing partner will probably want to seek a partnership post elsewhere and need a reference. It is only fair to tell the individual the type of reference they might expect: this will depend upon the specific reasons for and nature of each resignation.

Effects of breakdown on the partners

The reaction to a partnership breakdown or resignation will depend upon the events that led up to it. If all partners have tried to discuss and resolve differences it will be easier to come to terms with than a decision that is announced without warning. Of course, each individual will respond in a unique way and much will depend upon their viewpoint and the length of time that they have been working professionally with their colleagues. A partnership split has often been likened to a marriage breakdown and partners are likely to experience a similar range of emotions. If the partnership has divided into smaller groups there will be some mutual support and opportunities to review the sequence of events in detail. This may be enough to help individuals come to terms with it, and strengthen the new partnership. However, if one partner is ostracised they may not have a natural source of support or a de-briefing forum. If the practice has a strong manager they may be the person in whom everyone can confide, although it should be remembered that they will be coming to terms with their own feelings as well. Time must be given to allow all parties to reconcile themselves to new working arrangements to enable them to accept what has happened and move on.

Effects of breakdown on the practice staff

When a partnership runs into difficulty and subsequently dissolves the staff will be directly affected. When any partnership splits the position of the staff should be researched and agreed before any announcement is made to them. Quite naturally their first questions will be about the security of their employment or potential redundancy payments. The temptation is to underplay the upset by offering reassurances, when a clear statement of their position will be more helpful. Employment legislation can be complicated and any partnership considering dissolution would be well advised to seek a professional opinion from ACAS, a solicitor, the BMA or a medical defence body. If staff are going to be made redundant it is only fair to allow them the maximum time possible to seek alternative employment and offer time off to attend interviews.

If the staff have been with the practice for some time they may also need help to come to terms with what has happened. Here the agreed policy statement is invaluable and someone in authority should reiterate that it is a partnership decision and does not reflect upon the staff. Partners should try to behave in a responsible manner and keep their personal opinions to themselves, wherever possible, observing the common courtesies to maintain an atmosphere in which people can go about their normal duties.

SUMMARY

Partnership conflicts are no different to those experienced by any other team. The consequences can be greater given the financial implications and commitment to staff and patients. If a partnership consciously works towards improving communication and fostering an atmosphere where varying views can be openly debated, the conflicts will be contained and harnessed to positive outcomes.

REFERENCES

Hasler J C et al 1991 Handbook of Practice Management. Longman Group
Flew R 1995 onwards Organisational models. Various lectures and presentations in the old Oxford Region where Dr Flew is an Associate Adviser.
Martin P & Nicholls J 1987 Creating a Committed Workforce. Institute of Personnel Management

6. Conflict with practice management

There are any number of job titles for managers in general practice, each emphasising the priority of the post or defining the level of responsibility. In this section we will use the term 'manager' or 'practice manager' to describe the whole group and range of personnel undertaking the senior management role. They are the highest paid members of the ancillary staff and central to overall financial and organisational success – or failure!

In this chapter we will be taking the manager's perspective of general practice and looking at the inherent difficulties and idiosyncrasies of this unique position. All of the methods for preventing conflict with staff are applicable to the ways in which partners treat their practice managers.

General practice has increased, and continues to increase, in complexity. The practice manager's role has also developed, sometimes by a conscious policy decision with the approval of all partners and sometimes by default. The practice manager equates most readily with the managing director of a medium-sized private company. He or she must possess skills in administration, finance, personnel, information technology and strategic planning, and a working knowledge of all relevant legislation. Harder to quantify but equally important are maturity, common sense, tact, sensitivity, resilience, self-motivation, high personal standards, approachability, decisiveness and flexibility. A competent manager can enhance and strengthen a practice, a poor one can destroy it.

The flexibility of a manager is tested daily as the level of responsibility and authority is constantly moving.

- In terms of conditions of employment the manager is identical to any other practice employee and is protected by the same legislation.

- In decision-making the manager usually participates fully in business meetings and can offer valuable comments which are on a par with those of the partners.
- When changes and decisions need to be implemented the manager acts as a buffer between staff and partners. They have to translate policies into practical plans and motivate the team to comply.
- When policies have been agreed the manager is responsible for monitoring and maintenance. In this instance he or she is in charge of the whole team, including the partners, and upholds routine discipline (see Fig 6.1).

The ability to fulfill this ever-changing role will depend upon each individual manager's maturity and confidence. A new manager will take time to 'grow' into the job and feel able to exercise routine discipline over the partners, or to bring a contentious issue into the open at a practice meeting.

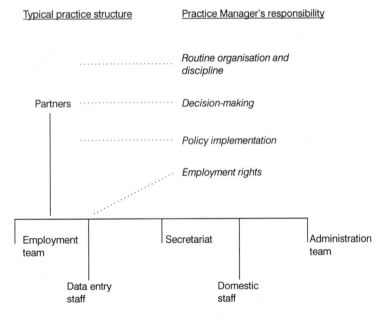

Fig 6.1

CLEAR REPORTING PROCEDURES

If the average manager is asked how many job descriptions he or she has, the answer will be in direct ratio to the number of partners.

Each principal assumes that the manager will adopt and further their personal interests: these could be anything from increasing partnership profits to supporting local businesses. Unwittingly, a manager gets caught up in conflicting priorities and, because arguments between partners swiftly become personalised, is labelled 'for' or 'against' certain people. This, of course, is grossly unfair as the manager will be trying to follow their own job description and offer an evidence-based judgment. In these circumstances the manager's effectiveness is compromised, largely due to the polarisation of the partners' feelings and unnecessarily strained working rapport. The longer-term impact is the manager's confidence becoming undermined and a refusal to tackle emotion-provoking problems.

To create a healthy working environment and to gain greatest value from managers, they must be allowed to manage. This is a difficult change of attitude for partners who have always been very involved in, or responsible for, the management of the practice.

Example:

Brenda works for a single-handed GP. She joined as a receptionist, was promoted to office manager and is now officially called 'Trainee Practice Manager'. Brenda is attending management training and is still paid at her original receptionist hourly rate. She is given full responsibility for every activity, except finance. The GP gets annoyed if anyone opens the quarterly Health Authority statements and keeps all of the ledgers, including salaries, at home. He has refused to promote Brenda and pay her accordingly even though she is fulfilling the management role as he wishes it.

The manager's remit need not be wide when they, or the post, are new. The important message to put across is what the manager is expected to do without reference to the partners, when they should consult the partners and what is clearly not their mandate. The natural place to look for this guidance is the job description, although it does not give specific parameters, e.g. any incidental expense over £50 must be authorised by the partners (see sample job description).

Sample job description

PRACTICE MANAGER
The Practice Manager shall be responsible for the efficient, effective and safe administrative and financial management of the practice; ensure the well-being of patients, doctors and staff and the successful, smooth running of the practice.

The Practice Manager shall have specific responsibility for:

PARTNERSHIP SECRETARY

The Practice Manager shall act as the Secretary to the partnership

- compiling the agenda for all the practice business meetings;
- convening, attending, participating and minuting all practice business meetings;
- convening, chairing and minuting all staff meetings;
- all financial controls and reports;
- confidential partnership matters, e.g. Partnership Agreement, retainers, contracts, partners' drawings;
- all administration regarding the local Health Authority or Commission;
- liaison with the practice accountant and any other professional consultant.

THE PARTNERS

- involvement in organising the out-of-hours duty rota;
- the instruction of registrars or medical students in practice management topics;
- personally supporting the partners in areas of practice management, as may be required;
- liaison with partners nominated to have executive responsibility in areas of practice organisation, personnel and management;
- monitoring doctor cover to maintain agreed minimum numbers;
- reminding partners of agreed practice policies;
- facilitating regular audit and clinical meetings;
- assuming the role of personnel manager to the partners;
- arranging an extraordinary partnership meeting if an important issue arises that cannot wait until the next planned meeting.

THE STAFF

- ensuring proper working conditions with respect to health, safety and welfare;
- securing and maintaining an efficient and cost-effective level of staffing;
- maintaining current job descriptions and contracts for all staff;
- holding regular performance interviews with all staff;
- maintaining an appropriate level of discipline;
- conducting effective staff training and personal development plans;
- communicating all practice policy decisions that affect working methods to all staff;

- ensuring that all staff understand and uphold the confidentiality of patients, partners and colleagues;
- assuming the role of personnel manager to the staff.

THE PATIENTS

- dealing with all patient complaints and liaising with the relevant doctor(s) to seek a satisfactory solution and follow the complaints procedure;
- monitoring standards outlined in the Patients' Charter, auditing and modifying systems as necessary;
- bringing all patient concerns and comments to the attention of the partners.

GENERAL ADMINISTRATION

- compliance with all statutory regulations;
- compliance with all legal obligations for employers;
- reviewing and maintain comprehensive insurance policies for buildings, computers and equipment;
- security of property and personnel;
- maintaining adequate stocks of all consumable items, e.g. stationery, couch rolls, disposable gloves etc;
- maintaining high standards of hygiene throughout the premises;
- maintenance of the buildings, gardens, car park and overseeing a refurbishment programme;
- devising protocols for data entry and computer systems management;
- devising systems to include all the data collection necessary for effective clinical and organisational audit;
- involvement in the business planning of the practice;
- maintaining effective and open communication channels between all sectors of the practice team.

FINANCE

- compiling and presenting budgets and targets to the partners for approval;
- administering the partners' drawings;
- maintaining accurate records of all items of income and expenditure;
- comparing practice item of service performance against national averages;
- administering staff salaries and salary review policies;
- timely submission of accounts for non-GMS work;
- cash flow forecasts and financial planning;
- reviewing methods of income generation.

STRATEGIC PLANNING

- keeping up to date with current NHS guidelines and advising the partners of any actions they need to take to comply with regulations and recommendations;

- attending training seminars appropriate to the future needs of practice management;
- assimilating new information, researching it and presenting it to the partners for their consideration;
- taking an active role in the development and direction of the practice as deemed appropriate by the partners.

PUBLIC RELATIONS
- arranging all practice functions;
- responsibility for all visitors to the practice;
- arranging regular informal gatherings of the practice team.

CONFIDENTIAL MATTERS

The Practice Manager must maintain and protect the confidentiality of partners, patients and staff at all times.

The Practice Manager may choose to delegate some parts of the role, but remains responsible for the actions of anyone acting on such instructions.

The Practice Manager will deal personally with all confidential matters that concern an individual partner or the partnership as a whole. There may also be other duties considered by the partners to be properly the responsibility of the Practice Manager that are not included above.

RECRUTING A NEW MANAGER

There is a growing trend for practices to seek outside help when they identify the need for a manager or wish to replace one who has resigned, retired or died. The external assistance may be in the form of a commercial recruitment agency, the Health Authority, an experienced local practice manager or a management consultant. The interesting point is the acceptance that the manager's role is crucial to the future of the practice and that few doctors feel totally confident in their ability to interpret business skills and translate their application into general practice. Perhaps the driving force to seek external input is the realisation that all general practices can take advantage of traditional commercial management competencies and the promotion of a senior receptionist or other in-house candidate will not enhance or develop the role.

The first step in the recruitment process, identifying a comprehensive job description, is fundamental in securing the right manager and is most often overlooked. To avoid partnership disagreements when a new manager is appointed the partners must decide the priorities in advance. Without a job description there is no benchmark or standard against which candidates can be compared.

Finding a new manager is not a cosy or informal sequence of events, it is a decision to invest in excess of £20,000 in terms of salary and training every year. As mentioned previously, a practice manager's post is attractive as the details of responses to a recent advertisement demonstrate (Box 6.1).

Box 6.1

Full-time Practice Manager	
£25,000 per annum	
in mid-Norfolk.	
Total enquiries	134
Total applications	78
Analysis	
Male	52
Female	26
25 to 30 years	6
30 to 40 years	28
40 to 50 years	35
Over 50 years	9
Backgrounds	
Bank or Building Society	6
Armed Forces	7
NHS –	
not practice management	9
practice management	3
Information Technology	5
Out of work	7
Other	41

When seeking a new manager a target start date must be clarified, as to go through the various stages correctly and allow for sufficient discussion at the significant points takes at least four months.

Stages in recruitment

Identify the need

Every vacancy is a positive opportunity to move closer to longer-term ambitions. A SWOT analysis of the management of the practice is a useful way to identify key priorities.

Agree job description

It is helpful to contact local managers and the health authority for sample job descriptions. It is easier to adapt an existing job description than to start from scratch.

Analysis of skills and competencies

From the job description a list of skills can be clarified, with some that are likely to be needed in the future.

Advertising

An advertisement is a means to attract candidates. Here quality is more import than quantity and the ad should convey a clear but simple message about the main skills that will be needed and major responsibilities. Box ads are more eye-catching (and more expensive) than lineage ads.

Responding to enquiries

To enable each candidate to have enough information to assess their own suitability for the post, it is a good idea to send out a 'package'. This would include the job description, practice brochure, brief overview of the practice and anything that will discourage unsuitable applications.

Pre-screening

Comparing the applications to the job description and analysis of skills and competencies. Identifying an initial short-list for interview. It should be remembered that only technical skills and experience can be judged from paper.

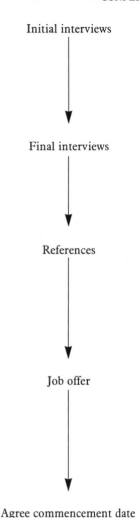

Initial interviews

At this stage the task is to verify the written application and confirm that the candidate can fulfill the requirements of the post. it would be usual for two partners to undertake the initial interviews on behalf of their colleagues.

Final interviews

A final short-list, of a maximum of four, to be interviewed by the entire group of partners. Here the personality traits can be explored and assessments made about each individual's style of management.

References

These should always be taken up before any appointment is made, and they should be written if possible. A telephone conversation can be helpful however, as previous employers may make verbal comments that they would not commit to paper.

Job offer

A verbal offer and verbal acceptance is a contract, but these should always be followed by written confirmation. It is a good idea to send a contract or conditions of employment with the job offer to enable any problems to be resolved before the person starts work.

Agree commencement date

New manager joins

If the successful candidate is employed in a management capacity elsewhere they will have to give at least one month's notice.

Good manners!

In the recruitment process partnerships are inclined to forget that the they are also being assessed by the applicant. Simple courtesies will enhance the practice reputation and create an image of a caring and well-organised unit:

- always acknowledge applications;
- keep candidates informed about their progress and the outcome of their application;
- always thank candidates for their time and interest in the practice.

Induction

It is unrealistic to expect any new member of the team, including partners and managers, to be effective from day one without some form of help.

This is most easily provided by a series of attachments to existing staff and health authority staff. The period of time involved need not be long, about a week is ideal to meet the whole primary health care team and find out the details of their roles and responsibilities.

On my first day at Calcot Medical Centre my name was on the office door, a 'welcome' card and a vase of flowers waiting on my desk. Apart from typifying the caring nature of individual partners, it started off our professional relationship on a very positive note.

LHC

The average practice will have executive duties for each partner. This system gives the new manager points of contact to discuss, and learn about, everyday issues. The educational process never ends and this type of contact should not be deemed unnecessary after a certain period of time.

APPRAISAL

Regular and honest performance review is as important for the manager as the rest of the staff, although the objectives may have wider implications. It is a normal management duty to ensure that annual appraisals are conducted for each member of the ancillary staff and that the partners are informed and consulted but not necessarily directly involved. In fact, few doctors would claim to have the skills to appraise their practice manager. This probably explains why appraisals rarely happen or are manager-led. Managers need feedback and not just the reactive variety in response to a crisis. Appraisal offers the partners an opportunity to take a balanced view of the manager's strengths and weaknesses, identify training needs and discuss the future development of the role, culminating in a set of personal goals for the coming year. This can reflect the need for training to tackle new initiatives and unresolved management problems.

At the end of each calendar year a practice must submit a business plan to the Health Authority, including bids for development monies. It is logical to appraise the manager in January when the practice objectives have been set. The interview can take the format of a structured discussion led by one or two partners who have been empowered by their colleagues. This will motivate the manager, who will gain a clear sense of direction and be able to enhance the ethos of the organisation. Complicated forms are not essential, although the manager's job description can usefully be updated to incorporate additional responsibilities.

TRAINING

There can be a somewhat unrealistic expectation that a competent manager will be able to respond positively and successfully to every challenge. To develop existing skills and acquire new ones, a doctor would consider regular education sessions quite normal, yet this attitude is not always extended to the manager. If anything, their role is more complex and continuously evolving so the need for training is imperative.

At the moment there is no qualification in practice management that will guarantee competence. The combination of business, financial and people skills would suggest at least three learning paths. The professional practice-management bodies all offer training courses to attain a certificate or diploma. Such courses need a commitment from the individual because the amount of personal time needed to complete assignments and do background reading will be great. Also, they are not cheap and it would be reasonable to expect some contribution from the practice, in the form of either funding or study time or both. The beauty of a modular training programme to be assessed for National Vocational Qualifications is its work-related emphasis. Practices who sponsor their managers will see the new skills and competencies demonstrated by improvements to routine activities and initiatives. The intention is for all parties to benefit.

DISCIPLINE

Many partnerships delegate disciplinary issues to the manager and remain on the sidelines offering advice and support. For this reason doctors do not maintain a working knowledge of employment legislation and disciplinary procedures, and normally would have no need to. Hence, when a serious problem occurs they feel threatened by their own lack of belief that they can deal with it correctly. Some partners adopt the ostrich approach and bury their heads in the sand, other rush in blindly and make mistakes that may result in a claim for unfair dismissal.

The manager's role affects every member of the practice team and the overall quality of care delivered to the patients. When a manager's personal conduct or performance falls below the required standard it must be dealt with promptly. Failure to do so can be misinterpreted, i.e. it can seem that the partners condone the behaviour. The routine enforcement of standards that a manager implements for the ancillary staff team is rarely echoed by the partners' attitude towards the manager. This is not an obstacle for practices who nominate a partner to liaise on all management issues. The partner and manager develop a rapport and by routine dialogue monitor the manager's performance and behaviour. For the manager it is a method to obtain personal feedback, a sounding board for ideas and, above all, a means to combat the inherent isolation of the role.

MANAGEMENT STYLE

Each manager develops their own management style to suit their personality and experience. Irrespective of the quality of training received, it will only be effective if the manager adapts theory to practical application. General practice is not a perfect environment to manage when there are no clear aims or reporting structure, added to which, some partnerships are unwilling to allow their managers to manage. Yet the manager's personal style can either minimise conflict or actively provoke it.

One common style can be summed-up in the phrase 'anything for a quiet life'. If it is taken to an extreme it can result in the manager being submerged by stronger personalities or bypassed completely if a tough decision is needed. Potentially difficult issues will be avoided at all costs as the prospect of dealing with the resulting upheaval and conflict will be too daunting. Most managers who find themselves repeatedly working in this way usually recognise it and wish to become more assertive. With support from the partners and training this can be achieved. When a reserved manager moves into a more pro-active style there will be some resentment from the team, who have evolved their own 'unofficial' hierarchy and methods of problem-solving. The transformation may be difficult in the short term, but has immense benefits in the longer term.

The reactive manager is the type who spends most of his or her time dealing with crises. They never behave as though they are in control as their energies are channeled into solving other people's problems. The reactive manager can be helped considerably by learning planning techniques and delegation skills. Some managers thrive on feeling that they are needed and actively encourage staff to bring them their problems. This is unhealthy for two reasons: firstly, the manager's time is poorly utilised and secondly, the team's acceptance of responsibility for their own actions steadily declines.

Lack of confidence or self-esteem may result in a manager simply implementing the partners' wishes and constantly looking to them for guidance. There are many possible reasons for this style of management – lack of permission from the partners to do otherwise or personal lack of interest. Complete absence of management input into the practice policy-making process is dangerous as the partners may decide that the manager is superfluous. In this scenario the staff are unlikely to use the manager as anything other than a means to pass their comments to the partners. The solutions for this style of management will depend purely upon the reasons and these can only be uncovered by an appraisal discussion.

Managers promoted 'through the ranks' are often unwilling to jeopardise their previous relationships with colleagues by taking a firm lead in the shape of unpopular decisions. This may be aggravated by partners who do not alter their own response to the individual's new status. An example would be the partners who expect a manager to cover holidays on the reception desk, or type referral letters when the secretary is away. The motivation to change this style of management must come from the manager himself or herself. It will be a slow and steady process using every opportunity to point out alternatives and clarify the role. A meeting with the partners to define authority and expectations would be useful, especially if the job description has not been reviewed for some time. The strength of such a manager will be their detailed knowledge of every member of staff, and this can be enhanced if domestic issues are not given priority over business decisions.

A consultative style of management is ideal as it allows for full and open discussion about all aspects of the practice and harnesses differing views to produce the best course of action. The potential for negative conflict is reduced as the whole team has been involved in the decision-making process. This does not mean that the manager cannot take a firm line that may be contrary to the wishes of the majority, but a consultative approach will foster respect and credibility.

Of course, no one works purely in one mode. A mature manager will use the management style that best suits any given situation, although every individual develops a norm that fits his or her personality, level of authority and circumstances of the practice.

THE EFFECTS OF A STRONG MANAGER

It would be the desire of many partnerships to enjoy the advantages of a competent manager. This assumes that qualities like loyalty and the best interests of the practice are present and paramount. Unfortunately this is not always the case and the effects of strong management can be benign or malign.

Malign effects

There are some basic sensible measures that partners can take to protect themselves, and especially their finances. Whilst it may be expedient to have the manager as a cheque signatory to avoid the partners being disturbed to sign cheques when they are busy, it removes a vital verifying step. A dishonest manager has unlimited opportunity to defraud a practice, usually because the partners have abdicated their responsibilities. We are all familiar with the partners who will sign any cheque placed in front of them without question, or worse still, sign a blank cheque. The manager knows the balance of every bank account and orders all of the equipment and consumable supplies, like stationery. All partners prefer to believe that their manager is scrupulously honest, and indeed, 99.9 per cent are; yet they do not maintain systems to protect both themselves, the manager and the staff. These need not be elaborate or cumbersome, just routine precautions. They could include making two partners responsible for checking all expenditure and bank reconciliations, restricting signatories to partners and maintaining a petty-cash ledger. When dealing with dishonesty prevention is definitely better than cure and any partnership which suspects any member of staff of mishandling money or property should contact their defence organisation for advice.

The other major malign influence can be harder to quantify and prevent because it centres around power and personality. When a competent manager has been in post for some time they will naturally attract and enjoy the respect of both partners and staff and they may unwittingly, or deliberately, become the driving force in the practice. This is not a problem if the manager consults the partners appropriately and works to achieve the agreed objectives. The influence becomes dangerous when it is abused and used negatively.

Example:

Grace has been practice manager for nearly 20 years and has enjoyed an excellent relationship with the partners. In the last year the two senior partners have retired and their replacements want to be more involved in management of the practice. One is keen to increase the profitability and the other wants to improve efficiency with sophisticated computer equipment. Grace feels very threatened and perceives their questions as criticisms. She starts scaremongering to the staff, claiming that any major changes will result in redundancies. Gradually all the staff turn against the new partners and resist any suggestion they make. Grace claims that she cannot understand the hostility of the staff and counsels the new partners to do nothing until the tension has disappeared.

Insecure and inflexible managers have a greater tendency to this type of behaviour as they can use it to hide their shortcomings and prejudices. Again, open discussion is the only way out of this pattern or possibly an away day to minimise the manager's power by agreeing the way forward for the whole team.

Benign effects

To give an impression that managers are constantly looking for ways to undermine or embezzle their partners would be false; the effects of strong management are essentially positive. The NHS reforms to create a purchase/provider split did not begin by offering general practitioners a budget by accident. They were perceived to have the necessary management skills and infrastructure to deal with the complexity of the task. This is a very visible indication of the value placed upon management and the opportunities open to competent managers to facilitate change and bring a strategic planning dimension to general practice.

Michael Drury defines management as a process of decision-making, involving seven elements:

1. Establishing objectives.
2. Defining roles, tasks and procedures.
3. Establishing priorities.
4. Securing and allocating resources.
5. Securing compliance.
6. Monitoring performance.
7. Watching the environment.

These neatly describe the functions of management that are translated into specifics in a job description, but they are not exclusive to general practice management. The functions apply to any organisation and are not necessarily undertaken by just one person. The larger the business the greater the numbers of people needed to manage it, the narrower the areas of responsibility and the more general management skills decrease. One of the biggest distinguishing features between a manager in industry or commerce and a manager in general practice is their relationship with their employer.

The manager is ideally placed to watch the behaviour of every member of the primary health care team and to step in where there appear to be problems. These are not confined to work-related issues and many managers undertake a pastoral role. As a manager becomes more established in a partnership they acquire a wealth of personal information about the partners, both domestic and financial. They will also be aware of professional aspirations and special interests. If a manager is approachable and sensitive to others he or she will perform a vital, often unrecognised, service, that of 'the listening ear'. Allowing individuals to let off steam in a safe environment can prevent disgruntlement growing into conflict, and the manager can move the problem into the open to gain some form of resolution by a variety of routes.

Examples:

The newest partner realised that on two days each week he was the only doctor taking 'extra' patient consultations and home visits. On these days he was working at least two hours longer than his colleagues. He was becoming increasingly tired and resentful. The manager knew that the other partners would be unsympathetic as they had all been in this situation when they first joined the practice. He arranged an audit of workload and outside commitments and raised the item at a practice meeting.

Simon's wife had just prematurely given birth to their second child; unfortunately she and the new baby were quite ill and kept in hospital. Daily enquiries by the manager about their progress highlighted how worried Simon was and the difficulties in arranging child-minding for their first child. Simon refused to take any time off, claiming that the practice was too busy. The practice manager called the available partners together and explained the situation. Simon's colleagues divided his workload between them and insisted he take the week off. Longer term a provision for paternity leave was added to the partnership agreement.

David was obviously feeling stressed; he had started to behave entirely out of character, was irritable and snappy, and everyone was giving him a wide berth. The practice manager went into his consulting room at the end of his surgery to see if anything could be done to help and to try to establish the cause of the problem. It transpired that there were some marital difficulties and the manager persuaded David to seek advice from his own GP.

These scenarios imply that a manager has a counselling role, and in some cases this may be true. However, amateur counselling is unsafe and normally starts with the phrase, 'If I were you ...' The manager's responsibility is to identify potential problems and guide individuals to seek appropriate professional help – avoiding home-spun advice along the way.

CAREER OPTIONS

A highly trained manager is a valuable commodity in any business, but historically practice management has been a non-progressive post. Recently there has been a growing trend of greater mobility between practices with managers moving to larger units to take on new challenges. The reasons for wishing to move may be simple ambition or an unresolved conflict about salary, recognition and contribution. When a manager leaves a practice to take a similar job elsewhere the partners would be well-advised to analyse objectively their view of management. It can provide feedback that is invaluable when seeking a replacement to ensure that history does not repeat itself.

Another innovation is to offer a manager partnership status, and there are several models already in operation. The Red Book does not recognise anyone other than an approved principal as a partner in general practice. Yet there is nothing to prevent a manager being given a vote on policy issues or being paid on a profit sharing basis. Using profit sharing is a motivational technique used by a number of multi-national companies. It links the manager in a more tangible way to the progress of the practice and encourages an objective view of expenditure. The pitfall is the danger of putting financial considerations above all else, but this can be countered by a fair basic salary with a profit-based bonus. The alternative is a salary review at the end of the financial year with the manager's increase in direct proportion to the profits. This would include no increase at all if the practice and partner's drawings have remained static.

In summary, the management of a practice is central to its success. The manager's role is complex and should be the subject of regular appraisal and review. To compensate for the lack of career prospects the partners must allow for the role to evolve and encompass new challenges and responsibilities.

REFERENCES

Hasler J C et al 1991 Handbook of Practice Management. Longman Group
Drury M and Hobden-Clarke L 1994 The Practice Manager. 3rd edition, Radcliffe
   Medical Press

7. Conflict with other health professionals

INTRODUCTION

Much of the conflict that we experience in general practice is generated from our own working group of health professionals, some of whom are employees and some of whom are specialist colleagues. Many of the disputes revolve around levels of responsibility and funding, so much so that we need to remind ourselves occasionally that everyone is endeavouring to achieve the same aim – the care of the patient.

In this chapter we will be reviewing each group of health professionals that a general practitioner regularly comes into contact with to fulfill their patient obligations. It will include the other members of the primary health care team and some aspects of secondary care, like hospital consultants.

CONFLICT WITH CONSULTANTS

The roots of the many differences between consultants and general practitioners date back to the Medicine Act of 1858. This divided the profession into three parts: the physicians, the surgeons and the apothecaries. The apothecaries, the forerunners of today's general practitioners, kept the provision of primary care, with referral rights to secondary care, while the physicians and surgeons retained secondary care and the hospitals as their domain. These differences, decreed by an Act of Parliament 139 years ago, mean that our patients need a referral letter prior to gaining access to secondary care. It also explains some of the ill feeling concerning the perceived threat of consultant-run open-access clinics and the advertising of consultant services.

From a working point of view most of us have reasonable relationships with many of our local consultants. We write our referral letters, the patient gets an appointment, gets seen and we get a letter back informing us of what action has been taken. There are a number of areas during that process where problems can arise and conflict can occur. Failure of communication has been cited before as a cause of conflict and it can occur between professionals as well as between us and our patients. Poor referral letters are often wrathfully quoted by consultants as examples of poor general practice. One-line letters that give the consultant little clue about the patient, and his or her needs and wants are very unhelpful. They may not only alienate the consultant from you but may set the wrong tone for the consultation with the patient. Equally, it is important for the consultant to tell you what they tell the patient. There is nothing more disconcerting than a patient coming to ask you what the consultant has said when the letter you have received says little about what the patient has been told of their diagnosis or prognosis. Some hospitals have standard format referral letters which may solve some of the problems but if these do not exist it may be worth working out a joint protocol which lays out the favoured content of both referral letters and their replies.

We refer patients to secondary care for many reasons. We refer for diagnosis, for investigation, for procedures and for relief. Sometimes we just need someone else to see a particularly difficult or complex patient. Unfortunately it is usually the very patient who will not benefit from another secondary care consultation who ends up in that situation. Typically this is a patient who has been well investigated but who fails to realise that his or her problems are psychopathological rather than purely physical. These patients often see the consultant as the person who is going to provide a cure for their physical symptoms at last. They have unrealistic expectations of the consultation. The GP and the consultant may also have unrealistic expectations which can be very

> I remember a young man of 28 with chronic neck pain. He had been thoroughly investigated and was left with intractable pain. Both he and I had unrealistic expectations for the future. I and his consultant kept looking for ways to improve his life and referred him to increasingly specialist units for advice. The consultant and I came into conflict over the management of his pain and it was not until we both saw that we were being manipulated that we could resolve the disagreement and help the patient come to terms with his situation.

difficult to address. The medical profession wants to help and it can be very difficult to resist further investigation just in case something very rare may have been missed. Rarities seldom occur and often the process of investigation will reinforce the physical symptoms and make it even more difficult for the patient to come to terms with their psychopathological condition.

Use and abuse of the system is not uncommon. We all know examples of chronic patients who become 'acute' on Fridays or just before holidays. Often this is because of the need to escape from an intolerable situation or because access to any form of respite care is limited. Nevertheless using the system in this fashion creates conflict not only between the consultant and the GP but also potentially between the patient and his or her carers, be he or she in a hospital bed or at home. There is no easy solution to this problem. Chronic care facilities are often scarce or very under-resourced. Sometimes discussion can get the consultant and social services on your side but all too often you are 'piggy in the middle'. Negotiation may prove a way forward in this sort of situation. Planning with the relevant caring agencies an emergency strategy for such crises may avert the need for the acute admission.

Funding is an issue that has created lots of discussion. Budgets are no longer as flexible as they once were, perhaps rightly so, and costs are being apportioned accordingly. Some conflicts have arisen over the prescribing of some new and very expensive medications. Hospital budgets do not have the funds to pay for these drugs and managers feel that the costs should be transferred to the GP budget. However, the matter of clinical responsibility must be considered. What doctor wishes to prescribe a new drug about which he or she knows relatively little when in doing so he or she assumes full clinical responsibility for that prescription? The consultant knows most about the area for his or her speciality and having recommended such a drug should take the clinical responsibility for prescribing it. Most conflicts arose when this first started happening and many such matters have now been negotiated sensibly, but with the continuing discovery and introduction of expensive new medications such problems will continue to arise.

We touched on resources earlier but they continue to be an issue which can cause conflict. Lack of beds, lack of time and lack of staff all cause inordinately long waiting lists both for outpatients and investigation and the problem does not appear to be getting any better. Inevitably the conflicts occur between the general practitioner acting as the patient's advocate and the consultant who receives the referral letter. Both parties have different pressures with which to contend and in the current climate of financial restrictions there are rarely easy answers. It is important to try and see each other's point of view and to appreciate that there are pressures on both sides. The general practitioner is under pressure from the patient and his or her family to get the problem seen to and sorted out at soon as possible. The consultant has to weigh the problem of limited resources, the urgency of the case and the priority of the others on the waiting list. There is rarely a correct or easy answer but conflict will be more easily managed if we understand each other's limitations.

Why does conflict between patients and consultants occur? Very often for the same reasons as we discussed in Chapter 3, such as failure to communicate, failure to listen and stereotyping. Although there is increasing teaching in communication skills at medical school and for those training to be general practitioners there is little such training for those working in secondary care. Budding specialists are trained in an adversarial environment where the patient is often seen merely as an adjunct to a pathological process and not as a human being with feelings, expectations and desires. No wonder then that we can all think of one or two consultants whom we respect as fine clinicians but who have failed to develop any communication skills.

Handling the situation of the patient who is upset or unhappy with the consultant to whom you have referred them requires great tact and diplomacy. It is easy to take sides but this is often inadvisable as you are only being presented with one half of the story. Listening and offering time to allow the patient to express their concerns is often all that is needed. If the patient is particularly angry encouraging them to write either to the individual concerned or to the hospital management may also help defuse the situation. It is likely that, whatever happened, the patient is going to be unwilling to see this consultant again and you will be involved in a second referral. It may be helpful to document the patient's

> I remember a situation when a patient returned to my surgery in tears complaining that the consultant had been rude and aggressive to her. He was known to be a bit abrasive at times and I defused the situation by allowing her to let off steam. I subsequently re-referred her to a colleague who knew the situation and chatted with him over the 'phone about the reason for the second referral. He was most understanding and all was well.

expectations and concerns in that second letter and so avoid whatever misunderstanding triggered the previous episode. It may also
be useful to discuss the situation with the second consultant prior
to the appointment just to remind him or her of the sensitivity of
the situation. This may resolve the situation for the patient but does
not solve the problem of a consultant with poor communication
skills. None of us practice in isolation and we all have some responsibility for our colleagues. In situations like this we owe it to our
colleague to tell him or her that the consultation went wrong. There
is no need to make any judgements but a brief explanation of the
facts as you know them may prove helpful. Most doctors do not like
upsetting their patients and some reflection upon the situation may
help avoid the situation recurring.

Fortunately there are fewer Sir Lancelot Spratts around today
than there were twenty-five years ago. We must recognise that
rather than each group acting independently, primary and secondary care can be seen as interdependent; we need each other to
provide the best possible service for our patients.

CONFLICT WITH COMMUNITY TEAMS

This section will address some of the issues that may arise when
dealing with staff employed by the community trust or health board
on the one hand, but who may be deployed into the community at
the request of the practice on the other. The situation is perfectly
designed to produce conflict not only from the team members' point
of view but also from that of the practice's and locality managers.

Commonly seen members of community teams are District
Nurses, Health Visitors, Midwives and Community Psychiatric
Nurses. There are other members of the team but they are less frequently seen in practice, for example, dieticians, occupational therapists, clinical psychologists and speech therapists. This section
will deal with situations affecting the more commonly encountered
members of the team but the principles of dealing with conflict in
this situation can be transferred to situations involving the less
well-known members of the team. Although the underlying causes
of conflict are similar to those listed elsewhere some are particularly evident in this group of professionals.

Most community staff only work in a particular practice for certain
sessions; their main base is elsewhere. This part-time presence can
lead to communication problems between attached and permanent

staff. These can be as simple as how messages are passed, how to arrange to discuss a case or, more seriously, clinically significant information or arrangements for clinical care may go awry. Such mischances will hopefully be relatively insignificant but they may cause aggravation for the patient, the member of staff or the doctor. Aggravation causes ill feeling and constant problems will certainly cause conflict to arise. Because of the particular communication difficulties attached staff have, some method of assuring communication and liaison should be developed within the practice. Perhaps a nominated member of staff could liaise or perhaps a message book could be used to make sure information gets passed on.

Belonging to the practice team is a good way of developing relationships and avoiding failures of communication. People who do not 'belong' remain outsiders and do not see themselves as members of the team. They do not function as part of the team and are a potential source of conflict. If attached staff are to 'belong' to the working practice team they will need to become valued by the whole practice. Membership means more than attending meetings, it means being kept up to date about the development of the practice and perhaps having a greater say in how their abilities can best be used. Having these professionals as part of the practice team may pre-empt further problems.

As community staff are employed by an agency outside the practice, they are required to follow the rules and regulations of their employing authority and to practice according to that authority's guidelines and protocols. This may cause conflict when the team member has to treat one of the general practitioner's patients. It is not uncommon for District Nurses or Health Visitors to undertake work in the practice on behalf of the general practitioner. The practice may have carefully drawn up guidelines for the procedure yet if the employing agency has a different set of guidelines, to which is the nurse or health visitor to stick? They are likely to have to adhere to those of the employing authority otherwise they may not be insured if something goes wrong. This causes some difficulty for the practice: having a set of guidelines is not much use if some of the staff cannot adhere to them.

Resolution of this issue can be difficult but it is important to be aware that it is not the fault of the attached member of staff. He or she is only obeying his or her employer. To solve the problem will require negotiation with the responsible manager and through him or her with those who developed the guideline or protocol in the first place. In a situation that you feel is potentially dangerous you may be obliged to ask the deployed staff not to treat a patient, but hopefully a working compromise can be reached.

All of the community team members are professionals in their own right. Nurses, Midwives, Health Visitors, whatever speciality they have followed, carry their own indemnity. Long gone are the days when the nurse was the doctors' handmaiden: we all work in a multi-disciplinary field with each of us having different skills in different areas. Some areas of care are effectively being removed from the general practitioner and are becoming the responsibility of others. Midwives wish to assume the responsibility for more and more ante-natal and puerpural care. Health Visitors undertake increasing amounts of developmental screening to the extent that some doctors are becoming de-skilled in these areas. It may be pleasant to have some of your work undertaken by others but de-skilling is a real risk and can cause conflict between the various professionals.

Having a strong, trustworthy and productive practice team is the best way of preventing conflict between the various professional members. Opportunities to talk, negotiate and progress should be provided and hopefully all your conflict will be constructive.

CONFLICT WITH FUND MANAGEMENT

The ethical and moral arguments about purchasing patient services are well documented and they inspire passionate reactions. The majority of personnel within the health service are 'pro' or 'anti' fund-holding; very few are indifferent. Even if the change of government in 1997 results in an abolishment of fundholding it will be replaced with another scheme, the most likely being locality commissioning.

The view of the partnership is irrelevant if all of the partners are committed to the same course of action and common objectives can be pursued. The conflict occurs when the partners are divided in their opinions and the decision is made by majority vote. The arguments are covered in more depth in Chapter 5; here we will confine ourselves to the ways in which the fund management team are affected.

Traditionally a doctor has made a choice to refer a patient based upon clinical evidence that has been explored during a consultation. The basic threat of fund management is that fund managers will interfere in this process and use financial constraints to restrict clinical care.

A practice cannot decide to take a budget without approval from the Health Authority and Regional Office of the NHS Executive. One of the criteria that has to be adequately demonstrated during the preparatory year is the management capability to manage a budget safely and within the given guidelines. The management can be provided in a number of ways – a partner or a practice manager extending their role, a newly appointed fund manager or a combination of a partner and manager. There is no hard and fast rule and the emphasis is on skills, not people. To compensate a practice for the costs of management and doctor time, amongst other things, there is a management allowance.

Before a decision can be made about the best option to manage a fund the responsibilities and duties should be defined in a job description (see example below).

Sample job description

FUND MANAGER

To liaise with, and be directly responsible to, the partners of the practice and to manage the fund efficiently and effectively.

BUDGET SETTING

- to provide all relevant information to verify budget offers;
- to liaise with the Health Authorities in the event of a difference between activity and budget offer.

MONITORING

- to enter all relevant patient contacts that form part of fundholding into the computer software;
- to follow all Health Authority guidelines and recommended data collection guidelines;
- to produce timely end of month statements and reports;
- to complete all statutory monitoring reports;
- to check performance against anticipated levels and advise partners of any discrepancies;
- to train all staff involved in fundholding data entry or data collection;
- to undertake regular patient surveys to assess quality standards;
- to participate in primary health care team discussions about the needs of the practice population.

CONTRACTING

- to attend all meetings to discuss contracting arrangements with providers;
- to be a positive part of the negotiating process and represent the views of the partners;

- to make all necessary information available to other members of the practice team involved in the negotiating process;
- to monitor activity levels and equality standards specified in existing contracts;
- to obtain the best possible financial and quality package to secure the patient services required by the partners;
- to obtain and keep up to date information about alternative provider prices and services.

MANAGEMENT

- to adhere to all the guidelines in the Manual of Accounts;
- to be involved in formulating practice policies to encompass fund-holding;
- to create and audit systems to support all fundholding activities;
- to advise the partners of the budget position at the end of each month, i.e. overspends and underspends;
- to take an active part in any local consortium groups;
- to facilitate audit meetings that have a direct impact on the budget, e.g. prescribing habits, practice formulary;
- to check each invoice in detail and liaise with providers in the event of discrepancies;
- to maintain effective communication channels between the practice and consultants, providers, other fundholding and non-fundholding practices;
- to facilitate fundholding protocols, e.g. lists of preferred consultants and units;
- to research the present potential innovations for discussion with the partners;
- to be available for any visitors to the practice who wish to discuss fundholding issues;
- to devise and maintain a mail protocol to ensure that the appropriate information reaches all partners of the practice;
- to undertake regular training sessions with the practice team to encourage their individual contributions to the fundholding process;
- to train a back-up team of staff to cover for sickness and holidays in the fundholding team.

TO BE RESPONSIBLE FOR ANY FUNDHOLDING OR RELATED ACTIVITY THAT THE PARTNERS DEEM TO BE PROPERLY PART OF THE FUND MANAGER'S DUTIES.

The process of designing a job description will facilitate discussion and help to quantify the amount of time needed to do the job. It will also make clear the competencies required to compare against current personnel. If the chosen route is to recruit a fund manager the selection process is the same as for a practice manager. The difference is in the conditions of employment because such staff are funded from the management allowance and their employment must be reviewed annually. Without fundholding their post becomes redundant and few practices can afford two managers.

The temporary nature of the position will affect the number and type of candidate as well as the partners' attitude to the appointment. They may be more willing to compromise on the basis that the person will only be with them in the short term and they can use the annual contract renewal to get rid of them if things do not work out as hoped. It is likely that they will seek specific financial skills and place less emphasis on team and communication skills. (Some may be more devious and actively seek qualities and abilities that the existing manager does not possess, rather than tackle a problem.)

The fund manager cannot work in isolation and interacts with the whole primary health care team. We will review each type of contact in turn.

The partners

If the practice is divided about holding a budget the fund manager will be the embodiment of the 'pro' camp and vulnerable to inappropriate criticism from the 'anti' camp. Rather than raise their views and concerns with their partners, by whom they have been out-voted, they will target the fund manager. The reactions will range from open hostility and lack of co-operation to complete lack of interest. Each extreme shows the partners' unhappiness and feelings that have not been properly addressed.

If the fund manager holds regular meetings with partners to discuss spending to date, waiting times and comparative prices at local providers, it may be perceived as pressure to put financial considerations ahead of patient needs. The fund manager may simply be trying to make the best use of the hospital services budget by seeking value for money. If the quality issues are considered to be equally as important as the financial ones and discussed at the same time, this potential conflict can be overcome.

When it comes to negotiating contracts with providers the fund manager needs the mandate of the partnership. Ideally the whole team will have shared their views on services that need to be improved and devised a list of priorities. These are likely to be quality issues, possibly in response to patient feedback. The benefits of fundholding have been in improved communication and an ability to match services to patients' needs.

The practice manager

When a practice has a fund manager and a practice manager the situation requires delicate handling. Clear job descriptions and designated areas of responsibility are essential, as failure to establish these basics will result in a power struggle and acrimony is guaranteed. There is a belief that fundholding can be 'bolted-on' to the practice and kept quite separate. This is true about pure data entry and the financial reconciliation of the budget, but fundholding will inevitably impinge upon practice systems.

Pre-fundholding:
The mail arrived each morning and was taken to the practice manager's office, where it was opened and sorted. Letters about patients were put into each doctor's tray immediately.

Post-fundholding:
The mail was taken to a central point and opened by the fund manager who sorted it into trays for the practice manager and doctors. All letters about patients that fell under a fundholding activity and would be chargeable were copied and the originals then placed in the appropriate tray.

Even this simple example of sorting the daily post has several points of friction:

a. The practice manager may resent this task being moved to the fund manager because access to all the mail is a method of keeping fully informed and following up partners.
b. Mail that arrives addressed to partners, but should be dealt with by the practice manager, may be placed in the partners trays and left unactioned.
c. There may be a delay in getting letters to the partners.
d. Copying may be delegated to a member of the practice team with a knock-on effect to their workload.
e. The practice manager may lose the social benefits of being the focal point each morning.

The fund manager may have been engaged on a higher salary than the practice manager. Some practices justify this by claiming that fund management requires special skills, like accountancy, and that they are only on a short-term contract. Irrespective of the explanation, in the practice manager's mind salary will equate to value. The partners may be faced with raising the practice manager's salary to be on a par with the fund manager's or receiving barrage of criticism every time the fund manager makes a mistake. Ideally, the fund manager will be aware of the delicate balance that has to be achieved and concentrate on forging good working relationships from the outset. Regular meetings, both formal and informal, between the two managers to discuss the most effective and least disruptive ways to integrate fundholding needs into practice systems is one method of avoiding misunderstandings and confusion. New guidelines to staff and training sessions will cascade the information to the whole administrative team.

The one area where practice and fund managers must liaise is the staff budget. This is a significant portion of the total fund and has to be monitored alongside the expenditure on hospital services, drugs and community nursing. At the beginning of each financial year there must be discussions about known turnover, relief cover and salary reviews. These can be turned into monthly targets and checked. Then, if the budget shows an overspend joint plans can be made to get it back on course.

The relationship between the practice and fund managers can be extremely positive and an opportunity for mutual education. It may combat the feeling of isolation felt by many managers and develop into reciprocated support. Visible signals of a strong professional relationship will deter staff from trying to manipulate the situation and pursue their personal agendas.

The practice staff

The fund manager has to maintain a working relationship with all of the administrative, secretarial, reception and nursing staff to gain the necessary information and feedback. To secure compliance, the staff need a basic understanding of the principles of fundholding and the scope of the scheme. An initial training session will allow for fears and questions to be addressed and give the team confidence to answer any patient's questions. When data is actually being collected and entered on the fundholding software and modifications to existing procedures are necessary, the staff should be consulted. The practice manager may prefer to undertake this role alone or in conjunction with the fund manager. The staff may have unrealistic expectations of the fund manager's level of authority and try to involve him or her in practice issues that are not within the remit of budget management. If this happens a fund manager is advised to guide the person gently but firmly to the practice manager or a partner.

The community nursing team

When the fundholding scheme was extended to include community nursing it empowered GP fundholders to delve into some quality aspects of their community services. The conflict with community nurse management is covered as a separate topic in this chapter, but the liaison between fund managers and individual Health Visitors and District Nurses merits a special comment. The first, and perhaps most surprising, reaction from community nurses was a desire to be employed by the practice rather than a community trust. This has never been allowed under the NHS fundholding guidelines and has never, therefore, come to pass. The perceived advantages were clearer reporting lines, the stability of working with one group of patients and the elimination of the 'employed' and 'deployed' dual allegiance. Many community nurses welcomed general practice input into the development of their role, their training and the skill mix of the team. The fund managers are ideally placed to strengthen links with the community team by improved communication and evaluation of workload.

The introduction of fundholding for practices who wish to go down this path has been invaluable. We have seen a general widening of management skills available to partners and the satisfaction of influencing secondary care. For the fund managers and data entry staff, the future has always been uncertain because their salaries are dependent upon the availability of the management allowance. This is an unsettling influence and many fund managers have actively pursued a career in practice management, seeing the wider remit of a practice manager as more attractive and more secure.

CONFLICT WITH TRUST AND HOSPITAL MANAGERS

Fundholding, total purchasing and commissioning practices have been in greater contact with hospital and trust managers since 1991. In the early days of fundholding this was a largely adversarial position, with general practitioners and fund managers trying to resolve long-standing secondary care issues. For some, it was their main reason for holding a budget. There is little doubt that the power base had shifted and primary care was able to influence secondary care in a meaningful way for the first time since 1948.

Those practices who opted to hold a budget were faced with a daunting task, but one that had potentially enormous rewards in improving patient services. The point of contact is between trust contracting manager, departmental business managers and fund manager, with parallel contact between consultants and general practitioners. The former is a financial and contracting forum, the latter a clinical forum. Both have improved the understanding of the other party's situation and constraints, although it has not always been a trouble-free process.

Looking back from a fund manager's perspective, the initial conflicts were about quite basic quality initiatives. For example, persuading outpatient departments to allocate individual appointment times rather than block bookings that could result in some patients waiting hours before they were seen by the consultant. This seemed a very straightforward change to GPs but it was interpreted as an implied criticism of the way that outpatient departments were organised. Indeed, in many cases it was. Another major debate was the insistence that a consultant see the patient for an initial assessment, not a more junior doctor who would simply arrange for the patient to be seen again if he or she was in doubt about the best form of management or surgical procedure. With general practice suddenly paying for all outpatient contacts, these situations came to light. Each required a change in consultants' work patterns if they were to be resolved and for this reason met with stiff opposition. Traditionally, secondary care had been led by consultants managing demand at their own pace. The concept of GPs interfering in this time-honoured regime and with the budgetary control to back their wishes was naturally met with disapproval and predictions that it would all end in tears.

Fortunately this state of affairs was relatively shortlived. Both trust managers and GP fundholders realised that if they could work together to improve services then several things would happen. By providing a better service each department would be able to attract extra referrals from fundholders who may have referred elsewhere in the past and the money following the patient would allow hospitals to expand their services by providing the funds to purchase new equipment or recruit additional clinicians. Instead of community hospitals being threatened, they were in many areas strengthened. If trusts could maintain consultant outpatient clinics in these outlying locations they would automatically retain any inpatient or day-case procedures at their main hospital. This was especially true when fundholders had a choice of main providers.

Some fundholders, with sufficient space within their premises, have been keen to expand the range of in-house services. Offering the facility to consultants to hold outpatient clinics at individual practices has been widely adopted. It is a win–win situation. The consultants and general practitioners improve their professional links via direct communication about individual patients, the clinic can be used as an educational opportunity to GPs if they are able to sit in, and the patients do not have to travel. This last point is of particular benefit to the elderly or those without private transport. The same principle has been extended to some direct access services like physiotherapy, speech therapy and chiropody.

It would be unfair to claim that the cause of all conflicts was the providers and their respective managers. Some fundholders had unrealistic expectations that could not be met and were not prepared to accept small but significant improvements at each year's contracting negotiations. The threat to remove their custom by referring their patients elsewhere was always the ultimate sanction and some fell into the trap of using cost, rather than quality, as the sole criterion for doing so. Indeed, many trust managers welcomed the financial drive offered by fund managers to seek improvements and fostered an atmosphere of liaison rather than confrontation.

The motivation for seeking to hold a budget predetermined the practice and fund manager's attitude to their providers. Those who were essentially satisfied with local consultants and hospitals and who enjoyed a good professional relationship with them probably entered the scheme to retain their freedom to refer to the person of their choice. This was particularly relevant for practices who used a wide variety of providers outside their region. Some were prompted by the need to tackle one or two departments, physiotherapy being at the top of almost every fundholder's 'hit list'. Others wanted to improve communication and retain responsibility for their patient's total package of treatment.

There were some less noble reasons for taking a budget, namely the prospect of making savings. If such savings are ploughed back into patient care by reducing waiting lists there is no moral dilemma. However, some practices have been allowed to use the monies to improve surgery premises if they fulfill the criteria. Understandably this was hard to justify to non-fundholders who saw NHS resources being moved out of secondary care and into GP's pockets. Large savings have steadily diminished as the budget setting process has become more sophisticated: this has been achieved by a combination of capitation-based calculations and more accurate data collection by fundholders and providers.

Fundholding arrived at the same time as the government's charter initiatives and a general uplift in the public's awareness of their position as consumers. Such published service aims fitted neatly with what many fundholders were trying to achieve: for example, a commitment that any patient waiting longer than 30 minutes beyond their appointment time to see a consultant would receive an apology and an explanation. Subsequently there have been league tables of hospitals' performances against basic criteria, like the amount of time a patient waits in accident and emergency departments before being assessed. Although emergency treatment is outside the scope of the standard fundholding scheme it forms part of the same push to improve services.

Annual contract negotiations have developed away from a pure activity and price basis to debates about quality issues. In most service agreements one would expect to see a clause about the patient's rights to privacy and full and clear explanations, and an insistence that they are treated with respect. This is to ensure that the ethos of general practice is extended into hospital care, as much as charter criteria. Some fundholders have initiated patient surveys on outpatient and inpatient contacts. A typical questionnaire would include the points shown in Box 7.1.

Box 7.1

Outpatients

- What was the length of time from GP referral to notification of an outpatient appointment?
- How long did the the patient wait to see the consultant beyond the given appointment time?
- Did the patient consider they had received enough information from the consultant?
- Was the patient given sufficient opportunity to ask questions?
- Were optional treatments discussed and explained?

Inpatients

- Did they see the anaesthetist and surgeon before their operation?
- Was the surgical procedure fully explained?
- Did the patient consider that they received sufficient attention from nursing staff?
- Comment on general hygiene.
- Comment on food, ambiance, visiting times and any other non-medical aspects of their stay in hospital.

This type of survey can be used to target one or two particular specialties where the fundholder perceives a problem, or can adopt a blanket approach to assess the overall standards.

One fundholder negotiating alone on behalf of their patients does not have as much power as several working together on behalf of a large group of patients: the activity levels and financial impacts are higher. Since fundholding was introduced there has been an element of liaison in geographical areas, reinforced by regular meetings with the Health Authorities. This does not mean that group contracts are compulsory, indeed, it is possible to negotiate shared aims together but contract separately, thus offering fundholders the best of both worlds.

Despite the resistance to fundholding and the claim that there would be a two-tier system, in reality a provider cannot cope with running two sets of systems. The improvement in standards has been across the board, benefiting all patients equally. When a fundholder invests more money to clear their patients on a surgical waiting list by paying for additional operating sessions, the remaining patients on that list have a shorter time to wait.

One fundholder's comment about the two-tier system:

'If we only had two tiers within the NHS it would be a dramatic improvement. There are currently any number of tiers as the quality and efficiency of each main provider varies, and GPs are at the mercy of the standards of their local hospital.'

When community nursing was included in fundholding, about two years after fundholding was introduced, similar conflicts arose between fund managers and community managers. Misunder-standings and misconceptions had to be overcome, also the culture change of having GPs influence skill-mix, staffing levels and recruitment. This aspect is covered in more depth elsewhere in this chapter.

The introduction of fundholding has been a prime example of the management of change within the NHS, and probably the most significant in its history. All the players started in the scheme to fight for their own agenda, equally determined that their view was the right one. Needless to say, this generated an enormous amount of unnecessary conflict at all levels. As each successive year has passed the extremes have been eroded, because the shared aim has been identified as the care of the patient. Once this has been formally established and the secondary and primary care teams realise the advantages of working together, the conflict disappears and in its place comes innovation.

8. Conflict with authority

In this chapter we will be looking at some points of conflict between general practice and authority. There are a number of bodies who govern what a general practitioner can, or cannot, do. These are referred to collectively as 'authority' and we will be examining the role of major players in the delivery of primary health care.

To understand the NHS, we must first understand its structure (Fig 8.1).

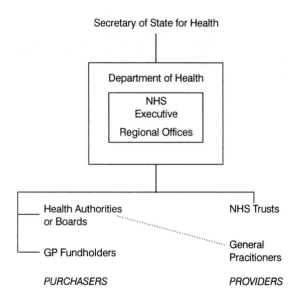

Fig 8.1

In April 1996 there was a radical restructuring of the NHS which resulted in the merger of District Health Authorities and Family Health Service Authorities to form Health Authorities or Health Boards. The Regional Health Authorities were amalgamated and became Regional Offices of the NHS Executive. It should be mentioned that we have used the model that applies to England; there are slightly different titles in Scotland, Wales and Northern Ireland, although the basic functions remain the same.

To assist the reader we give below a brief description of 'who's who' in the National Health Service:

Secretary of State
The Cabinet Minister responsible for the NHS.

NHS Executive
Responsible for setting the strategic framework for the NHS according to government policies and priorities. It is the head office within the Department of Health. The *Regional Offices* interpret the NHS Executive's decisions and communicate them to Health Authorities and GP fundholders. They are the arbiters in the event of a disagreement about budget setting or fundholding policies.

Health Authorities or Boards
These bodies are responsible for liaison with GP fundholders with regard to monitoring performance, budget-setting negotiations, training and routine queries. For all practices within their area they make the payments for all item of service claims, basic allowances, target payments, premises reimbursement and indicative staff and drug budgets. They monitor the statutory regulation of GPs, and deal with formal patient complaints and Patients' Charters.

General Practitioners
Doctors who have been approved to become a principal in general practice and who deliver primary care to their patients in accordance with their Terms of Service.

GP fundholders
Those practices who have successfully completed a preparatory year and who have been allocated, and accepted, a budget. They may be part of the standard fundholding scheme, community fundholders or part of a total purchasing pilot.

Providers
Hospitals or units which provide patient services following a referral from a GP or a nominated member of their team.

Community Health Councils
These were established in 1974 to offer the consumer a voice within the NHS. Their members are nominated by voluntary organisations,

local authorities and Regional Offices. Each Health Authority would have a Community Health Council. They do not have any specific powers but they do enjoy some rights to enable them to represent patients' views. These include the right to information and consultation, and to attend health authority meetings.

The Government has a dual role as purchaser and provider of health care. It buys services from the general practitioners who are contracted via the Red Book to provide primary care. It also sets targets for secondary care: an example of this would be that no patient should wait beyond a specific number of months for approved surgical procedures. The Government has a basic housekeeping problem – demand exceeds supply. The population is living longer, there are a growing number of elderly patients and medical techniques and treatments are getting more sophisticated, and inevitably, expensive. There is a finite amount of funding available to the health service, which means that there must be rationing. Each year we see certain procedures removed from the NHS and the only way that a patient can access them is by using the private sector: e.g. tattoo removal. To date these have not caused any controversy, mainly because the medical profession can agree to safeguarding resources by saving on cosmetic operations. What will happen if the exclusions become tougher as the Government identifies its priorities to contain expenditure?

The new GP Contract of 1990 was perceived by general practice as a means to make the profession work harder to achieve the same level of income. Certain health priorities were imposed, some without any apparent clinical benefit. The edict to weigh and measure the height of the over 75s at an annual medical examination was felt to have no medical validity – it was only a means to check if the patient had been reviewed – although it must be said that the introduction of targets for childhood immunisation and cervical cytology have had a very positive effect and the financial incentives have ensured that this type of valuable screening is comprehensively delivered. It is easy to sympathise with the cynicism of certain general practitioners; they have seen their workload increase, income barely keeping pace with inflation and little scientific evidence to support some mandatory clinical tasks.

We must think about the cost-effectiveness of the whole system, not just primary care. For example, long waits for cataract treatment can increase demand on community and social services when a patient has to be maintained in his or her own home. Similarly, long waits for relatively minor operations like hernias and bunions may result in additional expenditure on State Sickness Pay and employer's sickness benefit. A criticism of a health service that is under the control of the government of the day is the lack of longer-term strategies. We have seen too many instances of 'quick fixes' just prior to an election, and any plan is medium-term or until the next general election.

Understandably, general practitioners see themselves as the patient's advocate, not the gatekeeper or rationer of care. They are, however, contracted by the Government to provide medical care and these two roles come into conflict, especially when GPs are asked to police their patients. This can cause major conflict with the ethics of patient care. When there are requests for medical examinations that can have a huge impact on the patient's income, future employment or ability to drive a car, some practices insist that these are undertaken by a doctor other than the patient's own. To certify a long-standing elderly patient, who you know relies upon his car to maintain his independence, as unfit to drive may severely harm the patient–doctor relationship. It is better for a partnership colleague who does not have the same rapport to make the unwelcome decision, leaving the regular physician in the more comfortable position of commiseration.

The NHS has clearly defined the patient services that fall within General Medical Services, and there are recommended rates to charge for services that fall outside. Typical examples would be patients asking for passport photographs to be signed or applications for gun licenses. The perception of the public is still that a general practitioner's services are free of charge, irrespective of the reason. When the GP is aware of the patient's financial circumstances they find collecting fees very difficult, often waiving the charge altogether sooner than damage their relationship with that person.

Given the number of general practices who have opted to become fundholders, the profession seems to be divided in half in its attitude to taking financial accountability for services. Like all initiatives, fundholding is neither all good or all bad. There is little doubt that fundholding practices have had a significant effect on reducing prescribing costs, shifting the power base away from consultants and improving community services. There will always be moral dilemmas about big savings and the ways in which these can be spent. Fundholding has been well-received by practices who have a choice of providers or where there were on-going problems that control of funding could address. The disadvantage has been the administration costs, necessary to manage the budget safely and effectively, but removing funds from patient care. As the budget-setting process becomes more accurate, or as a result of capitation-based budgets, the potential for a fundholder to overspend is greater. One measure to bring a budget back on line is to put a temporary halt on hospital elective admissions, though this conflicts with the advocate role.

To leave the control of patient services in the hands of Health Authorities as non-fundholders continue to do is also an imperfect system. It would be naive to assume that a Health Authority can monitor individual patients through secondary care with the same accuracy as their general practitioner. The contracts that they agree are vast and monitoring is a purely statistical and accounting exercise, with data being provided by the hospitals themselves. The Health Authorities contract for the whole range of services, including those that are outside of a fundholder's remit. It is perfectly possible for them to run out of money before the end of the financial year, which would have a dramatic impact on essential services, like emergency care. The individual practice may not get its proper share of resources in a blanket contract.

Example:

The Health Authority contracted for 100 hip replacement operations for the locality. The Woodlands practice should have had 10 patients admitted if the contract had been allocated pro-rata. The provider made no distinction between practices, other than that they were either fundholding or non-fundholding, and performed the 100 operations by the end of November. Woodlands patients had only accounted for 2 of those hip replacements.

From this example it is easy to understand why non-fundholding practices have felt disadvantaged in the distribution of resources. It is hoped that the development of locality commissioning will address just this sort of issue. It will give non-fundholding GPs a voice and facilitate their inclusion in the negotiations between Health Authorities. To work together with a local group of practices with similar patient profiles and needs will offer power without the need to hold financial responsibility for a hospital services budget. There will inevitably be criteria to enter into such a scheme, but at the time of going to press these have not been published in a White Paper.

One ongoing bone of contention is the level of paperwork. In 1995 the Cabinet Office decided to order a scrutiny into bureaucracy within the NHS to see how cumbersome administrative systems could be streamlined. Many of the recommendations have been introduced, for example, the number of item of service claims forms has been reduced from 23 to 4. One of the overriding principles when a new system is introduced centrally is probity. Each Health Authority implements the system using their own interpretation of the guidelines; safeguards have traditionally been built in to avoid abuse. The introduction of computer links has gone some way to reduce paperwork and unnecessary form-filling. The Audit Commission also play their part, especially with regard to fund-holding practices. Anyone spending public money has to be publicly accountable. The Manual of Accounts, the budget management bible, has to be observed and certain documents compiled, retained and audited.

One of the appeals of being a professional is that society pays you what you are worth. It is not surprising that general practitioners feel undervalued by Government when they have to haggle over the percentage pay award each year. There is a levy on GPs to pay for the General Medical Services Committee (GMSC). This body represents all GPs via the Local Medical Committees (LMC). The GMSC presents evidence to the Doctors and Dentists Review Body (DDRB), as does the Department of Health. The DDRB in turn present a report to the Government, who are supposed to action it. The British Medical Association negotiates on behalf of the profession. Conflict arises when the Government, who appoint the DDRB, do not uphold its recommendations. Other branches of the medical profession work in the same way and put forward a case to the DDRB; inevitably someone is disappointed because the pot is finite.

The NHS restructuring of 1996 altered the relationship between general practice and its immediate governing body, the Health Authority. GPs had become used to the Family Practitioner Committee (FPC) role, which was solely administrative. The FPC officers were a source of advice on the Red Book and the organisation was seen as the paymaster. It was a harmonious liaison with few conflicts. When FPCs became Family Health Services Authorities (FHSA) the emphasis shifted as it became obvious that their brief from the Regional Health Authorities had been extended beyond administration. The FHSAs monitored compulsory submissions, like the annual report. They became involved in the purchaser–

provider split and their responsibility was to allocate and negotiate budgets with fundholders and contract for non-fundholders. Part of the remit was to implement the changes in funding for practice staff and introduce indicative drug budgets. As organisations they became far more innovative and evolved their role into a managerial one, although they continued to fulfill the administrative function. The introduction of cash-limiting prompted inevitable points of conflict, especially where direct reimbursements were concerned. The strength of FHSAs was their personal knowledge of practice teams within their areas and the personal rapport helped to overcome many of the difficulties. Now that FHSAs have merged with District Health Authorities they mirror the Government's position, that of purchaser and provider, with all the attendant complexities.

For all the criticism of the infrastructure of the NHS it still achieves the basic objective that essential care is free at the point of delivery to patients, irrespective of their means or circumstances. Rationing is a fact of life and expenditure on the health service is a big influence on the nation's economy. There will never be unlimited resources and we shall no doubt see a succession of schemes to reduce management and administration costs to put the additional money into patient services.

9. Finding the balance

PERSONAL FEELINGS AND ANXIETIES

Others
practice staff
partners
patients
spouse
children
lawyer
tax assessor
neighbours

Experience of life shows that, because, as individuals, we have differing needs, opinions, aims, and world views, we often find ourselves in conflict with others. 'Others' may be within our practice, within our family or within the social system in which we live. We have to deal with that conflict. We can suppress it, ignore it, react aggressively to it or perhaps we can use it constructively and move forwards.

Being placed in a situation involving conflict is usually pretty uncomfortable both psychologically and physically. Your blood pressure rises, your heart rate goes up and you get a dry mouth. You feel anxious. All these symptoms show that your 'flight or fight' reaction has been stimulated just as if you were about to face that sabre-toothed tiger back in prehistory. These reactions are quite appropriate when dealing with an escaped tiger or a short-term problem like a collapsed patient; they enable us to perform at a higher level of arousal and have all our energy and skills directed to helping the person on the ground (or running away from the tiger).

Although the body's reaction is appropriate if you are about to face the tiger or deal with the collapsed patient, the reaction becomes very draining if you have a long wait before putting your energies to use. If the conflict is prolonged, generally the effect upon us as individuals is fairly unpleasant. We become over-aroused and anxious. Our emotions become disturbed, relationships with those close to us can suffer and we tend to feel out of control and unbalanced. All this happens because our reaction to conflict has not been dealt with. We need to find some form of release that helps our bodies and minds unwind. For some that will be a session in the gym, for others a round of golf and for many sado-masochists (like my husband) a 10-mile run. All these help us manage the conflict; the result of mismanaged conflict, for the individual, is stress and it is as a stressor that it causes us most distress.

STRESS

What is stress?

Stress is a term used freely to describe almost anything. Definitions abound and it is said to cause the loss of thousands of days off work each year. Psychologists tend to think of the stimulus as the stress while doctors dealing with stressed patients define the response to the stressor as stress. Other groups have even more definitions for the word. It is perhaps best to consider stress as the end result of several interacting factors and responses working together.

This section may get a little technical so feel free to leap over it if you wish.

What causes it

There are many models of stress and its causes; the model in Fig 9.1 seems to explain the concepts sensibly and clearly enough for our needs. Those who wish for further details should refer to a detailed psychology text. In this model, *stressors* can be divided into three main types: cataclysmic stressors like an earthquake, the surgery burning down or other major disaster; personal stressors such as unemployment, bereavement or moving house; and background stressors or daily hassles with which we live all the time such as inconsiderate smokers, high noise levels or overwork. All these elements go into the stressor part of the equation and they are all

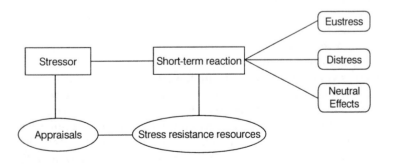

Fig 9.1   Source: Sheridan and Radmacher, *Health Psychology,* 1992)

weighted differently by different people – one man's (woman's) stressor may not be another's.

Fortunately, cataclysmic stressors occur rarely (how many earthquakes do you recall in Britain?) and because when they do happen so many people are in the same situation there are instant support mechanisms available as well as a large group of people with whom feelings and behaviour can be compared. Cataclysmic stressors tend, therefore, not to be such a problem as might be supposed. Personal stressors have been studied and their impact varies from individual to individual. Holmes and Rahe (1967) developed a 43-item life-event scale, grading such things as moving house, divorce, bereavement, and even taking a holiday, which has been extensively used to study the effects of personal stressors. Background stressors, the daily gripes and recurring problems of which we can all compile a list are potentially more draining and damaging than either cataclysmic or personal stressors.

The effect of all these stressors is influenced by how we look at them or how we *appraise* them. We appraise stressors in two dimensions almost simultaneously, firstly by their direct effect upon us: is it dangerous, is it good for us, is it neutral; and then we look at how we can handle it. Another factor in the stress equation, our *stress resistance resources*, affects both how we appraise and how we handle stressors.

Most of us survive in a world filled with stressors and psychologists suggest we handle them using all those things which we have available in our lives that allow us to cope (our stress resistance resources). These include income, food, clothing and shelter. Without these even simple tasks become very difficult and stressful, yet with them life, and the payment of bills, becomes relatively straightforward. Our bodies bring lots of resources to the equation, our fitness, attractiveness, our general health. Knowledge and education are positive stress resistance factors as is a sense of belonging to a social group or culture.

The *short-term reaction* in the diagram refers to the short-term biological effect the stressor has upon you, or how aroused you become to solve a problem. Increases in heart rate, blood pressure and glucose levels, as well as constriction of the blood vessels supplying the skin occur. Obviously these responses can be very mild or strong depending on the strength of the stressor.

The diagram shows three outcomes to exposure to a stressor. Some stresses are actually good for us and raise our performance to higher levels, *eustress*. Some have no effect upon us, the *neutral effects*, because either the demands they make are very small or we have plenty of resistance resources with which to combat them. *Distress* is the term used in this diagram to describe the adverse effects of being exposed to a stressor, in fact it is synonymous with the word 'stress' as used by many people including doctors. A multitude of things causes us distress: running late, a patient's unexpected death, having

> **Symptoms of distress (stress)**
>
> *angry outbursts*
> *aggression*
> *irritability or hostility*
> *tired all the time*
> *sleep disturbances*
> *increased levels of minor illness*
> *poor timekeeping*
> *poor judgement*
> *inability to concentrate*
> *memory loss*

a complaint made against us. All these stressors lead to the 'flight or fight reaction' coming into play and it is when this situation becomes prolonged that we see the development of psychopathology.

Stress and the health professional

Helping patients to manage their illnesses is good for the patients but it is a significant stressor to those who look after them. Not only do health professionals have to deal with the heavy emotional demands of their patients, but they must also deal with their own emotions and concerns. Unfortunately few health professionals look after themselves or even acknowledge that they can suffer from any illness, let alone a stress-related illness.

This failure to deal with stress-related illness has some unfortunate sequelae. Doctors, in particular, have a high level of marital problems, which often lead to divorce. Partnerships may break up because of stress-related issues. Additionally, doctors have a high incidence of drug and alcohol abuse, of psychiatric illness and of suicide.

Burnout

Burnout is a term typically used to describe a pattern of chronic distress seen in the helping and service occupations where the pressure to serve others is associated with heavy emotional demands. Burnout is defined as a syndrome of emotional exhaustion, depersonalisation and a feeling of reduced personal accomplishment. As emotional resources decline it becomes increasingly difficult for the carer to give of themselves at a psychological level, a tendency which leads to emotional exhaustion. The development of depersonalisation is characterised by negative feelings towards one's patients, cynical attitudes, the use of black humour to cope and apparent lack of caring in a caring professional. The third aspect of burnout, a feeling of reduced personal accomplishment, refers to the tendency to evaluate oneself negatively, particularly in relation to work with patients. The consequences of burnout can be severe; Christina Maslach's research showed it to be a factor in job turnover, absenteeism and low morale. It is also correlated with the same pattern of findings as described in those suffering from chronic distress: that is, personal dysfunction, marital problems and substance abuse.

Avoiding burnout means that stressors must be managed appropriately. In order to manage them we must be aware of what they are and from where they could come. We then have to discover or invent strategies that will allow us to reduce their impact upon our lives: we have to learn to cope.

Identifying stressors

Earlier in this chapter the need to use sources outside those of the medical professions was mentioned. The model that will be described for assessing the source of some of the stressors in our lives is based upon one developed by Rosemary Stewart, a well known writer in management theory. In this model she views the tasks undertaken by a manager as coming from a number of different directions over which the manager has varying amounts of control. By looking at these levels of tasking within a general practitioner's life we can see the sources of many of the stressors that impinge upon him or her. The model could equally well be applied to a practice manager and the analysis

Demands
• Boss-imposed
• Peer-imposed
• Externally-imposed
• System-imposed
• Subordinate-imposed
• Self-imposed
(after Stewart)

provided could give some insight into those areas of working life over which there is some control and where there is scope for negotiation or movement. There are many demands upon our time and resources, as health professionals, and the model helps look at the sources of these demands and put them into context.

As general practitioners few of us are in the situation of having *boss-imposed* demands; we work within a partnership but those new to the partnership may perceive themselves to be in the position of a subordinate and see the more senior members of the partnership as their boss. We have little control over the demands imposed upon us by a boss, whether those demands are real or perceived, and that lack of control is a potential stressor. The boss may define working practice and require adherence to protocols with which the new member of the team is not familiar. The boss has power, whether real or perceived, over our daily lives. However, we must remember that as general practitioners we are bosses to our employees. We have to think of our staff and think of how our demands affect the daily workload of our practice manager, our nurses and other staff.

As a member of the partnership is a member of a group of peers, there are therefore *peer-imposed* demands: demands of time and commitment, to be on call, to do the work for the journal club, to attend the monthly commissioning meetings and to attend the practice meeting regularly with a report about progress. All these commitments fill up our day and we need to be conscious of the time pressure they place upon us. We have some control over the demands placed upon us by our peers in that there is probably room for negotiation over the importance and priority placed upon these demands. It is worth reviewing these issues and rationalising your programme if at all possible. The practice manager may have no direct peer as there is usually only one practice manager in the practice. He or she also has no peer support so does not really escape the demand.

Many things we do, whether general practitioner or practice manager, are *externally imposed*, in fact our entire raison d'être is to serve external demands. Our patients and staff expect us to turn up on time and to be kind and pleasant to them, they expect us to be professionally competent, our families demand our time and resources, to collect children from school or the cubs, to attend plays and parents' evenings, or just to be with them and to offer quality time. Again we have limited control over *externally-imposed demands*. If we fail to stay competent we will lose our patients and quite possibly our jobs. If we neglect our family's needs we may well also lose them. However, some planning and negotiation may be possible and by managing our time efficiently we may manage to satisfy most of these demands.

System-imposed demands – the system within which we work places many demands upon us. These may vary depending on whether a practice is fundholding or not but will certainly involve attending meetings, filling in forms or perhaps developing proposals. The system constrains the way we work at times and that in itself places demands upon us when we are asked to work in ways that may not be wholly justified. Again control seems to be imposed upon us by the system but in this instance we have some power to delegate much of this work to others, for example, fund managers or practice managers.

We are employers, therefore we have *subordinate-imposed* demands upon our time and energies. Our practice manager may be the usual interface between the staff and the partners but staff need care and attention, if they are to perform well, which cannot all be left to the practice manager. Staff need appropriate training, regular appraisal, counselling or guidance; each individual will have different needs but these needs must be addressed if you are to have happy, functioning staff. Again, many of these demands should be, quite properly, delegated to your practice manager, however, you are also a manager and must be aware of the loads you place upon your practice manager: remember that he or she too is a subordinate who has needs.

Last but not least we have *self-imposed* demands upon us. We all have expectations of ourselves, most of them unrealistic! We expect to provide a high standard of care, we feel we should do lots of continuing education, we expect to be perfect parents, doctors and managers. These can often be the most difficult demands with which to cope as our expectations of ourselves are often far too high. Coming to terms with our own expectations is a challenge worth undertaking. A close look at what we do and why we do it may allow the redistribution of some of our resources.

The previous paragraphs have demonstrated that we all have a huge number of demands placed upon us some of which we have more control over than others. In order to find a balance, therefore, we must look at these demands and decide what is capable of achievement rather than what we feel we should achieve. If we do that we will end up successful, not in distress. It is a relatively simple process to document all the demands placed upon you in a working week or month – it is more difficult to prioritise these demands within the context of the practice and to decide what is achievable. Do you need to attend that committee every month? Has the practice manager got the time and resources to take over the fundholding accounts? Do you really need to employ another member of staff to take on several demands? At the cost of a slightly reduced income the number of stressors from which you and your partners may suffer may be substantially reduced. Planning how you handle all these demands may significantly reduce the number of stressors to which you expose yourself.

Coping with stress

The psychology of coping with life's stressors is worth briefly summarising. There has been much research done in this area and of necessity these few paragraphs are incomplete. However, they may give you some idea of the strategies we tend to use when faced with a stressful situation.

Coping with life's stressors involves using our stress resistance resources to overcome the short-term reaction caused by the stressor (see Fig 9.1). Psychologists suggest that there are three major components of coping, all of which are interrelated, and to cope effectively with a stressful situation all three components come into play. *Rationality* is defined as an accurate objective assessment of the stressor. If your reaction to a stressor is irrational, and you believe that a stressor will harm you even if it will not, your body will react as if your belief were true and will respond with the 'flight or fight' reaction. The converse is not necessarily true; if you do not believe noise is harmful and go to a very noisy rock concert your body may still suffer harm. *Flexibility* involves choosing the most appropriate coping strategy for the situation you are in. People who are not flexible cope with stress poorly: they either have a limited number of coping strategies available to them or are only willing to consider a small number of those available. Lastly, *farsightedness* is the ability to anticipate and assess the consequences of our coping strategies. Those who have an inability to be farsighted may find that the solutions to their problems are worse than the actual problems.

An alternative, yet related, way of looking at coping mechanisms looks at whether the coping can be classified as problem-focused or emotion-focused. Effective coping seems to require realistic and accurate assessment of the stressors and the available stress resistance resources; these are often undertaken in problem-based coping methods. Problem-focused coping not only involves the areas mentioned previously but also involves, practically, stress monitoring and the development of social skills such as assertiveness. Emotion-focused coping often involves reappraisal; the situation has not changed, it is just that the way it is interpreted that has changed. Avoidance and denial are also common emotion-focused strategies. Avoidance means removing yourself from the situation – out of sight out of mind – while denial means ignoring the stressor or explaining it away. Both methods of coping are effective in the appropriate circumstances.

The situation and how it is appraised seems to have the greatest effect on coping strategies, with those who believe that the stressor can be managed tending to use a more problem-focused style. This may explain why work-related problems tend to be handled using the components of rationality, flexibility and farsightedness.

Additionally, there is great variety in individual coping patterns. Differences in our stress resistance resources and the way we appraise a stressor probably explains most of the variation. However, personality also has a part to play in the equation, with 'hardy' individuals seeming to cope better with stress than the less 'hardy'. We all use different defence mechanisms to a lesser or greater extent and these too can alter how we cope with the stressors we come across in our daily lives.

Stress management – managing stressors

There is general agreement that the first step in stress management should be removing as many unnecessary stressors as possible from the equation. Some stressors are completely outside anyone's control, but some background stressors can be tackled at a personal level. Noise is a particularly significant background stressor. If your children constantly play their radios at full volume try and negotiate some quiet times during the day. If your practice lies on a busy main road perhaps investing in noise-attenuating double-glazing would make life bearable. Cigarette smoking is a stressor to non-smokers. In many places it has become policy that health centres are smoke-free zones: this makes life pleasant for the non-smokers and passes the correct messages to the patients.

Some of the most intense stressors come from working with other people. These can range from minor irritations to wholesale arguments. In the minor cases the solution may be straightforward; the individual may not be aware of the bad habit that annoys you, and simply discussing the issue may solve it. In the more serious case the conflict has to be managed differently and may require a third party to become involved.

Stress management – modifying appraisals

Our appraisal of the situation can have a significant effect on the impact of the stressor. A shy and timid receptionist may misinterpret a brusque comment from one of the doctors. This may cause feelings of inadequacy and insecurity, tears and a totally ineffectual receptionist merely because the doctor came to work with a headache. To avoid overreaction we must modify the appraisal of the stressors and look at them more rationally. In practice discussing your appraisal of the situation with an independent party may clarify the reality of your perception and bring the issue into proportion. Effective appraisal often involves setting priorities – we have to decide what is important to us and what is not. People who become over-stressed often magnify trivialities into major stressors which need to be looked at rationally and realistically in order to bring them into proportion.

Stress management – stress resistance resources

We use our stress resistance resources in order to help us cope with stress. There is increasing evidence that a healthy lifestyle aids us in coping with stress. This means that we should enjoy a balanced life of physical exercise, healthy foods, and an appropriate time away from work enjoying play. Regular exercise helps combat the draining effects of constant stress and a healthy body often produces a healthy mind. Our minds need a rest from our daily work and a hobby or pastime often offers a change of pace and refreshment.

Stress management – managing the stress reaction

Having accepted that stress, stressor or distress, exists and causes real problems for some people how should we manage the stress reaction? Psychologists use various techniques such as autogenic training, biofeedback training, progressive relaxation and meditation. The first two methods are quite technical and, apart from referring you to any good psychology or stress text, will be discussed no further.

Relaxation and meditation are both areas where we feel we can find out information. Most practices have access to a community psychiatric nurse who will almost always have access to relaxation tapes, many health food shops sell such books or tapes and they are quite straightforward to use. Almost every one is slightly different and uses a slightly different relaxation programme. The one you choose to use should be the one with which you are most comfortable. The example given here is only one of many.

Relaxation

1. Find a quiet place without too many bright lights.
2. Position yourself comfortably, preferably lying down on your back with toes pointed upward and palms up and arms by your side.
3. Close your eyes and listen to yourself breathe – begin to recognise each phase of breathing – in, hold, out, hold.
4. With each exhale tell yourself to relax; as you exhale let all your muscles relax; starting from the toes work up through the body relaxing each area in turn.

Because relaxation is highly sought after today many routes to that state have become available. The Eastern philosophies, yoga and transcendental meditation are all concerned with a way of life but some aspects of these philosophies, particularly those to do with relaxation, have been adapted so that they can be used within our society. As relaxation techniques these seem to have some beneficial effects in the management of stress.

Transcendental Meditation

1. Get yourself quiet and comfortable.
2. Close your eyes.
3. Turn your attention to your word – a mantra is often used.
4. Don't worry about your mind wandering: when you notice that it is, draw your attention back to the word.
5. You don't have to say the word, you can visualise it, imagine you can hear it, or even just be aware of it.
6. Take a passive attitude and observe the various changes that take place in your mind.
7. Try and do this for about fifteen minutes.

Some larger employers run stress management programmes for their personnel and, while this may be difficult for the average practice to arrange, possibly a session on stress and its management at the next practice meeting would be useful with an away day dedicated to the issue planned as a future event.

CONCLUSION

Stress (distress) is a recognised problem within many organisations today. It probably exists in your practice and in your life. We have seen that it makes people function less well and contributes to ill health. We all need some level of stimulus in order to function; it is when that stimulus becomes overwhelming that our performance declines. It is important that we look at our lives critically and see where we can alter our schedules and the level of demands placed upon us. We must all learn to say 'NO' and mean it. If you don't your inability to cope will become a problem for the family, the practice and yourself.

REFERENCES

Elliot-Binns C, Bingham L and Peile E 1992 Managing Stress in the Primary Care Team. Blackwell Scientific
Holmes T H and Rahe R H 1967 The social readjustment rating scale. *Journal of Psychosomatic Research*, **11**, 213–218
McKenzie C 1994 Perfect Stress Control. Arrow Business Books
Mulligan J 1988 The Personal Management Handbook. Warner Books
Open University Business School 1994 The Capable Manager (Workbooks and Texts). Open University
Sheridan C and Radmacher S 1992 Health Psychology. J Wiley & Sons Inc

10. Managing conflict

Conflict exists within every organisation and at any particular time there is likely to be a variety of different disagreements and conflicts within your practice. Managing conflict will very much depend on how you view it whatever your role. Is conflict something uncivilised which only causes problems or is it as a natural consequence of the differences that exist between the people in your practice?

One of the stereotypes of managers is that they thrive on the stress of conflict. No doubt there are those that do, but by far the majority of us find that dealing with conflict does not come easily or naturally. Conflict situations are threatening, they generate unpleasant feelings and make us feel uncomfortable. Consequently, we tend to view conflict as 'bad'. We see it as a symptom of deeper problems and as something to be avoided or suppressed at all costs. Unfortunately such attitudes often lead to disaster. Conflict is very real to those involved and avoiding it or suppressing it does not mean that it will go away. As the conflict festers it takes over a lot of the energy of those involved. The parties may demonstrate poor motivation towards their prime tasks and fail to co-operate with those seen to be on the 'other' side.

However, conflict can have benefits all of which would be lost if it were avoided or suppressed. Constructive conflict involving discussion or even argument about the design of a new medical centre may expose previously overlooked problems and may prevent them being built into the new premises. The process may be uncomfortable but if undertaken in a positive manner may lead to better interpersonal relationships and team building.

Conflict is normal, it is an inevitable feature of any organisation, whatever its size. It is a feature of people working together. Remember that it can be both constructive and destructive. This chapter will review ways of recognising conflict and then discuss some management strategies. The model used in this chapter is taken from 'The Capable Manager', a course provided by the Open University's Open Business School.

SOURCES OF CONFLICT

What kind of problems can cause conflict to arise? Mullins suggests that there are ten main sources of conflict within any organisation. Some of these do not apply to the area of general practice but the rest are worth reviewing.

Individual differences in perception

People are complex organisms made up of their beliefs, values, education and experience. They perceive other people and events from different viewpoints and often come to different conclusions. Ideally we would all recognise and understand these differences but in reality we live in a society where discrimination, prejudice and ignorance conspire to prevent understanding. Misunderstanding and misperception can create conflict.

Limited resources

Limitations in human or financial resources can be a major source of conflict within an organisation as individuals or groups compete for more resources than are available. Space and time are two resources which are usually fairly limited in general practice.

The interdependent nature of work activities

'No man is an island'. Within a practice all the work activities are interlinked. The efficient running of a surgery requires the office staff to select the correct records, the receptionists to allocate appointments correctly and the doctor to turn up on time. A failure in any one of these areas may lead to conflict within the practice.

Role conflict

People in organisations fulfill roles which are ascribed to then because of the work that they do. Consequently they are expected to behave in certain ways. If their behaviour is different to that which is expected conflict can occur. As a practice manager your role as the 'boss' can be in conflict with your role as counsellor or professional colleague. If your staff expect you to work on their behalf but the partners expect you to run the practice efficiently you can end up in a complex conflict situation.

Inequitable treatment

In dealing with employee rights or any reward system that might exist perceived or actual unfairness can result in conflict.

Violation of territory

People tend to become very attached to their own space, their office, their desk, or their seat in the staff room. They resent intrusion into that space or having it or themselves moved. When a practice moves into new premises there is inevitably some grieving over what was lost even if it was cramped. Allocation of new 'territory' has to be done fairly or it could lead to conflict over the move and the loss of personal space.

Environmental change

People tend to resist change because of the uncertainty it can engender. A move to new premises, the introduction of a new computer system, a change in the appointments system can all seem very threatening. Staff could react by trying to block the change or by making it difficult to implement. In the early days of computer systems in practice some 'old stagers' refused to use their terminals and caused conflict within their practices.

External disruption

Conflicts at work can be a consequence of difficulties in other aspects of people's lives. The sorts of conflict that occur in our family and social lives may spill over into the workplace.

Recognising the sources of potential conflict does not mean you can always stop it occurring, but being aware of the underlying cause may increase your self-confidence in handling it.

SIGNS OF CONFLICT

To deal effectively with conflict you have to recognise it. Usually the signs of conflict will be very apparent but sometimes they are less visible and lie underneath the surface of the practices' day to day life. Overt conflicts are easy to spot, those hidden behind the facade of everyday life are less so. Fortunately, although well camouflaged, even hidden conflicts usually have some tell-tale warning signs that might suggest that you look for underlying problems. For example, in a practice thinking about whether or not to become fundholding the doctors may divide into two factions neither of which can discuss the issue calmly and constructively. Overt signs of

> **Overt signs of conflict**
>
> arguments
> sniping
> rows
> raised tempers
> heightened emotions
> formal disputes
> disciplinary actions
> complaints

> **Signs of hidden conflict**
> coolness or formality in relationships
> uncomfortable silences
> issues which keep reappearing on the agenda
> unwillingness to communicate
> avoidance of sensitive issues
> down talking remarks from one to another

conflict such as raised tempers or an unwillingness to be helpful may be evident. With that problem drawing your attention it is often easy to miss what the problem is really about. In this case, it may be that the older partners feel very threatened about the increased workload of fundholding and think that it will be too much for them; as a consequence they may resist the move towards fundholding but because they do not wish to lose face they do not declare their concerns. The real problem may be well hidden but the conflict it creates makes everyone extremely uncomfortable. You must find the real cause or you may be trying to solve the wrong problem. If the real cause of conflict remains unaddressed or unresolved the situation may get out of control and at the very worst a practice split may occur. If things become sufficiently unpleasant the practice may even see itself making the medical press.

CONSTRUCTIVE CONFLICT

Conflict, when well handled, can often benefit both those involved and the practice. More productive interpersonal relationships, better group dynamics, improved ideas and working practices are all potential benefits. A prerequisite for constructive conflict, however, is an atmosphere of mutual trust and openness. Under these circumstances all parties feel safe enough to speak freely. Conflict is likely to be destructive if the groups within the practice are very closed and polarised.

Interpersonal relationships can be improved by giving people the room and the security to express any strong feelings that they may have about their colleagues and their job; this is much healthier than allowing these feelings to fester. Although we allow ourselves strong feelings about our own work, often we do not realise that our colleagues may also have their own strong feelings about their work. A sudden confrontation may lead to exposure of these feelings, which, while not a very comfortable experience, may lead to better understanding within the team.

Group dynamics are a feature of every group, including a general practice. We belong to many groups, the practice, the church choir and the yoga class. We have a role within each group and that role varies from group to group. Conflict can help the group function better by allowing personal agendas to be reviewed openly and by allowing the group to become responsible for its own development. Seeing colleagues actively disagreeing in a safe group situation may give permission to those who are uncertain of themselves to participate more effectively in the work of the group.

Finally, conflict often generates improved ideas and working practices. Conflict requires innovators to justify their ideas, so that the ideas get reviewed very carefully and may even be strengthened, alternatives may be considered and at the end of the day better solutions found. Conflict over working practices may reveal underlying structural or procedural issues that have been overlooked. Once these are corrected the entire practice will have benefited.

STRATEGIES FOR MANAGING CONFLICT

There are a number of strategies that you can use when faced with a conflict that you have to manage. But before deciding which strategy to use you will have to evaluate the situation. You will have to ask yourself some serious questions.

- How serious is the conflict?
- Does the conflict need to be resolved quickly or not?
- Is it a win–win situation or a win–lose situation?
- Is it just a trivial or healthy disagreement?
- What are your preferences?
- Have you the authority to deal with the situation?
- Have you the skills to handle the situation?

If the conflict is relatively trivial you may wish to observe it and let it run its course. If, however, there is any danger of escalation you will probably want to intervene. Remember, however that your perception of 'trivia' may not be the same as another's. The strategies that you may wish to use are conveniently grouped under the following five headings:

- ignoring;
- allowing;
- reducing or containing;
- resolving;
- preventing.

Ignoring

We all have difficulties in dealing with conflict. We tend to associate conflict with unpleasant feelings, anxiety, mixed emotions and general uncertainty. All of these are stressors and one way of avoiding them is to ignore them. If a conflict is genuinely trivial there may be no adverse consequences to ignoring it. However, there is a danger that the conflict may become destructive and by ignoring it the situation may deteriorate.

> It is easy to ignore two people who are sniping at each other. Ignoring the situation gives them time to work it out. That works if the situation is resolved but if others become involved you may required to take notice before the skirmish escalates into all-out war.

Allowing

If the conflict is trivial, likely to be short lived or seems to be constructive it may be appropriate to allow it to run its natural course. However, if emotions and feelings have become heightened, you may have to take some action to resolve the situation. Not only may you have to offer support to those involved but you may be required to help your staff explain their feelings and put the conflict into perspective. Participating in a conflict is a stressor and your staff may also need help in dealing with the feelings and anxieties associated with stress. Even if you feel that the conflict can be allowed to progress naturally you must maintain a watching brief just in case it becomes destructive and you need to intervene.

Deciding when, or even whether, to intervene is not easy. If the work of the practice is being hampered or the conflict shows signs of worsening you will probably feel you should do something, and the next section will look at some methods of intervention.

> You may allow a short-lived conflict over the mix up of duty nights to pass without interference. Such things happen and usually they blow over. It is not an issue unless it happens again. If the problem does recur, you may have to intervene because by then feelings have usually become aroused.

Reducing or containing

Strategies aimed at reducing or containing the conflict can be subdivided into short- and long-term responses. Short-term strategies can be used if something has to be done straight away. Although they may give some short-term relief, they do not usually solve the basic underlying conflict. These strategies rely on your position, power and authority to resolve the situation, and to succeed your practice team must both trust you and respect your judgement.

Short-term strategies

- *Persuasion.* People can sometimes be persuaded to call a halt to a conflict for 'the good of the practice' or because of the disruption it is causing among the staff. If loyalty to you or to the practice outweighs any potential gain from the conflict, you may succeed, but often the cause of the conflict is so deep-seated that the protagonist is unlikely to put your needs and interests above his or her own.

  If two members of nursing staff are being difficult over the allocation of a room for an afternoon clinic, they may be persuaded to halt their conflict. As the patients and the practice are the losers an appeal to the combatants may result in a truce.

- *Coercion.* People can be forced or coerced into stopping a conflict under the threat of disciplinary proceedings. Although this may work for a short while, the underlying anger may only be fuelled by the threat and the conflict is likely to recur with the additional difficulty that you are now part of the problem. If the protagonists' behaviour is disruptive to work, disciplinary action may become necessary. You must be careful, however, that the conflict is not just a symptom of an underlying problem and that the protagonist becomes a scapegoat.

  If two receptionists spend many of their working hours creating difficulties for each other, failing to pass on messages, not doing the filing correctly and generally disrupting the function of reception the threat of disciplinary action may cause pause for thought.

- *Buying Off.* Individuals can be bought off by offering them something they can get without conflict if they give up their battle.

  A young partner who is rocking the boat because he wants a clause added to the partnership agreement allowing a year's sabbatical may be bought off with a lesser expense such as a day release course which the practice might fund in order to retain his services.

- *Arbitration.* Under these circumstances both parties to the conflict present their case to you and using your authority you decide between them. You can choose one side or the other or you can develop a compromise. Unfortunately the loser will be very unhappy and often even a compromise solution will not last long. The compromise has more chance of success if you can really get the two protagonists to understand that this solution is the best and fairest of those available.

There is a long-standing argument about holiday allocation amongst your staff. Unfortunately all your records were lost when the computer crashed and two staff are arguing continually about the issue. Arbitration may work here although it is unlikely to create a win/win solution.

Longer-Term Strategies:

Longer term strategies may take longer to follow through but they are more likely than short-term ones to be effective if the conflict is deep seated. They do not always cure the conflict but they may help contain it and allow you to cope with the situation.

- *Separation.* Separating the warring parties may bring about peace. However, that is not always easy to do in small organisations such as general practice. This strategy works best if the problem is interpersonal conflict or if the conflict is limited to a few antagonists.

If the protagonists are part-timers it may be possible to arrange their working hours so that they do not overlap. If a branch surgery is in operation separating the two members of staff physically may also help. However, modern communications may work against you.

- *Mediation.* In mediation your role is to help the antagonists understand that each of them has an opinion which for each of them, at least, is valid. You may be able to mediate in a conflict within your practice but you may be seen as too close to the problem and as likely to take sides. In this case it is advisable to get help and employ an external mediator. A management consultant may perform this role.

In the event of two members of staff remaining in conflict over an issue which seems irresolvable and where neither appears to see the other's point of view, mediation may help. If you are too close to the issue an expert may help but if you choose to undertake the role yourself be prepared to listen actively to each side of the issue and without taking any stance try to get each protagonist to see the other's point of view.

- *Appeals.* For some types of dispute you may be able to refer a conflict to a higher authority. In some practices there is a mechanism whereby antagonists may submit their problem to a designated partner. For disputes over pay and terms of service formal procedures may be extant, for other scenarios special arrangements may have to be made. Not only may antagonists prefer the relative impartiality of a decision made by a partner but the threat of referral may concentrate minds and encourage the antagonists to look for solutions themselves. This will work in a practice with an active practice manager within the administrative structure. However, there may be difficulties in a small practice where a partner is also the 'hands on' manager who may have been directly involved in handling the problem: this is not an exclusive issue to general practice and is common to most small businesses.

If an issue reaches appeal, earlier attempts to resolve the issue have already failed. The conflict is probably deep-seated and you are in a difficult situation. Ideally you should not have been involved with the earlier attempts to resolve the problem but sometimes this is inevitable. It is important to document the process carefully and to be impartial in your judgement. Remember you may have to defend it at an industrial tribunal.

- *Confrontation.* If a conflict is simmering away causing unpleasantness and bad feeling it may be productive to bring some of these feelings out into the open. You could arrange a confrontation meeting where the antagonists can express their real feelings and perceptions about each other. This is a high-risk strategy, for individuals may refuse to co-operate, or, if they do participate, feelings may be aroused even further. Under these circumstances it is usual to employ an outside negotiator who is skilled in dealing with these situations. If the confrontation is successful however the pay-offs are high. A new atmosphere of openness, honesty and trust can develop within the organisation.

This strategy comes with a '**practice health warning**' as it can generate a lose/lose situation for all parties involved. If one party walks out in the middle of the confrontation, it cannot be completed. Worse still, the focus for all the conflict may switch to the practice negotiator and may close all avenues for resolution. This could lead to a disciplinary situation from which the practice as a whole loses.

Resolving

Resolving strategies tend to be longer term and aim to find a solution to the conflict. They not only deal with the present problem but also seek to promote an atmosphere where destructive conflict is less likely to occur. Individuals and groups within the practice may have different goals. In establishing common goals your aim is to get the members of the practice to set aside their own differences or at least put them to one side while they settle on higher aims for the practice. Sometimes the structure of the organisation lends itself

- Establishing common goals
- Restructuring
- Improving levels and processes of communication
- Integrative bargaining

to impose conflicting requirements upon different members of the team. In the situation of a practice with a branch surgery the staff working at that branch surgery may have different goals, quite naturally, from those working at the main practice site. In order to create unity amongst the practice as a whole it may be necessary to rotate staff through both premises so that they can see for themselves the needs of the practice as a whole, not just one subdivision.

Poor communication and understanding between individuals and groups of staff within the practice are likely to lead to polarisation of views and to the existence of groups with widely differing values: a potential starting point for destructive conflict. Good communication involves the breaking down of barriers within the practice and the establishment of communication networks at all levels. At an organisational level this may involve the staff learning more about the practice and what each individual contributes to the whole. Rotating round various jobs is the ideal way to give this breadth of experience. The aim is to promote good communication at all levels and to allow the development of a culture where anybody can ask for

Do not assume that you are at fault when Mrs Jones, your secretary, looks upset; ask her what the matter is. If the problem is work-related perhaps you can solve it. If it is a domestic problem, well, at least you can listen and share it with her.

clarification of an issue or can explore what others mean. Communication networks need to exist between staff at a personal as well as professional level. The culture of the practice should encourage communication at all levels. Good communication within the practice makes the development of conflict less likely.

A method of improving interpersonal communication during conflict

Aim: to structure a process between two individuals so that each can express their views without interruption.

Procedure:

- A is allowed to say what he/she thinks. B listens without interrupting other than to clarify matters of fact. A continues until he/she feels that B has listened and understood his/her point of view.
- The process is reversed with B talking and A listening.
- The process is repeated as necessary.

Integrative bargaining is a way of converting a win–lose situation into a win–win situation. Essentially, neither side in the conflict should have to give up any vital issue but both sides, working together, should seek a creative solution rather than a compromise. This solution should satisfy both parties.

Preventing

Perhaps the best way of handling conflict is to prevent it happening in the first place. Your staff and peers will always have differences; some of them will be superficial and some will be very fundamental. There are no guarantees that you will succeed but to try to prevent conflict you must encourage a climate where the practice team seeks win–win solutions rather than win–lose solutions to any conflict that arises within the practice. You are looking for an attitude of mind where people are willing to look creatively for win–win solutions; this kind of atmosphere is more likely to happen if communication channels are good and if your staff have open minds about the direction in which they are travelling.

By setting a good example we can demonstrate ways in which we can help our staff and improve the atmosphere within our practice.

Respect others and treat them as you would wish to be treated.
Only criticise in a constructive and friendly manner.
Do not make assumptions about people's feelings – check before you act.
Before altering someone's work reflect on whether or not their input would be valuable.
Positively reinforce constructive conflict.
Do not make or condone any attack either behind someone's back or in public.
Try and allow both parties to a conflict to walk away with some dignity – do not let them back themselves into a corner.

HANDLING CONFLICT

When you have to handle a conflict within your own practice, remember that from the moment you start dealing with the conflict you are a party to that conflict. How you are perceived will be fundamental to your ability to resolve the situation. You must reflect carefully on your own views and not make assumptions on their correctness until you have established the facts.

Be aware that the problem presented to you may not be the real underlying problem and it is likely that there will be many more parties to the conflict than is first apparent. You are unlikely to identify all parties involved until you begin to gather information so be very careful with whom you share that information. Be aware that any written reports are likely to be affected by the personal involvement of the author and may be sanitised to such an extent that they are of little value.

Ensure you use a four-stage process of handling the conflict – data collection, analysis of options, selection of preferred option and taking action – whether you elect to take a formal or informal approach. In any event, make sure you understand any legal implications and are briefed on the correct procedures before commencing any formal disciplinary action.

At all times, focus on the problem, not the person. Be prepared for that focus to shift and reveal multiple or layered problems, then make sure that you are absolutely certain of your facts. Expect to be briefed by your peers on their perception of the problem but remember they too may have a vested interest in directing you towards certain conclusions or a course of action.

Listen carefully to the reasons given for actions taken or attitudes and beliefs that are expressed; do not immediately dismiss them as irrelevant – they may be the indicators of the real or other underlying problems.

CONCLUSION

Conflict is part of our lives; it is part of working with people. As a principal or practice manager you will have to live with and manage conflict. A lot of conflict is constructive and healthy. It may lead to improved ideas and working practices, improved dynamics within your group or improved interpersonal relationships. However, if it is wrongly handled the converse may come about: reluctance to put forward ideas, lack of team work and a breakdown of interpersonal relationships.

Prevention is better than cure, and for conflict it is perhaps more accurate to say that accommodation is the best route. By creating the right working atmosphere the constructive element of conflict can be harnessed and utilised to best effect and the destructive elements can be dealt with as an everyday issue and not by creating drama from crisis.

REFERENCES

Mullins L 1989 Management and Organizational Behavior. (2nd edition) Pitman
The Open Business School 1994 The Capable Manager (Units and Texts). Open University.

11. Case studies

The reader is invited to think through each scenario before moving on to the suggested answers.

CASE ONE

> It is Monday morning and you are about to start a very busy surgery – there are already lots of extras fitted in! Will the morning ever end? First on your list is Mrs Patel. She has brought her eleven-year-old grandson with her to interpret.

Think through the potential sources of conflict in this situation.

Suggested answers:

- Forming a relationship when under pressure.
- Offering quality time when under pressure.
- Communication problems – language differences.
- Has the eleven-year-old got the words to explain his grandmother's problem?

> Mrs Patel is in her 60s, and moved to Britain five years ago. She now lives with her eldest son, his wife and family in a small, two-bedroomed house. She is attending for a routine check of her hypertension.

Any more issues that cross your mind?

Suggested answers:
- Mrs Patel was brought up in another culture with different expectations and health beliefs.
    - What does hypertension mean to her?
    - Is she taking her treatment?

- Is she seeking advice from her family at home and is she
  receiving any patent medications which could alter her
  clinical picture?
- How do I find out what is going on?
- How do I resolve the possible conflict between the two cultures?

**Her blood pressure is higher than normal so you try and discuss her
condition and her need for medication. Her grandson tells you that
his grandmother is fine since his uncle sent her some special medicine from home. Mrs Patel nods vigorously.**

Anything else?

Suggested answers:

- Mrs Patel is obviously taking some kind of proprietary medicine
  which may or may not be interfering with her antihypertensive.
- How to maintain a relationship while challenging her health
  beliefs? Perhaps an adult interpreter with an understanding of
  Mrs Patel's culture and health beliefs could help explain
  hypertension.
- Perhaps you need to compromise with her treatment.
- There are no right answers.

CASE TWO

**Now you are running 15 minutes late. Mrs McPherson walks in with
all three of her children. A riot ensues over your toy box. Mrs
McPherson moved down to the South from Scotland a couple of
months ago.**

Think through the potential sources of conflict in this situation.

Suggested answers:

- You are running late and everybody is being kept waiting – not
  good for relationships.
- A riot around the toy box is likely to make you annoyed and
  frustrated particularly if the mother shows no sign of controlling
  the children.
- New patient – need to establish a working relationship.

> Mrs McPherson starts explaining the problem to you in a very broad accent which you can barely understand. 'The wee one's been a bit girney over the weekend. She's caustive – nothing has happened since Saturday.'

What is she talking about?

Suggested answers:

- The problems of dialect exacerbating a difficult consultation.
- A frustrated doctor and difficult communication may lead to conflict.

> You eventually discover that she is constipated and you advise that she is given lots of fluids and some fresh orange juice. (She is two.) Mrs McPherson is obviously not happy and you try and find out what is wrong.

What do you think is wrong?

Suggested answers:

- Failure to meet patient's expectations – the mother expected you to prescribe a laxative to solve the problem and your attempt at health education did not work.
- Unrealistic doctor expectations – Mrs McPherson may also have problems affording fresh fruit juice which will make compliance difficult.
- Different health beliefs.

CASE THREE

> What a Monday morning! The next few consultations go fairly well, then you discover that the next patient has a very thick set of notes. Forty and female with lots of referral letters and lots of Lloyd George cards. The last thing you need this morning is a heartsink patient!

What kind of problems are you storing up for yourself? Think through the potential sources of conflict that could arise.

Suggested answers:

- You are stereotyping this patient before you ever see her and getting into a frame of mind that may not be receptive to her problems.
- Failure to communicate as consultation starts off on the wrong foot.
- Difficult to form a relationship when you feel so negative.

Mrs Johnson comes into the room with her husband. She is small slight woman. She tells you that she was at the hospital last week and they want her to continue on CPD (continuous peritoneal dialysis). She needs more dialysis fluids. Previously the hospital has provided these but they have sent her to her general practitioner as they will be unable to provide fluids in the future.

Where are the potential sources of conflict in this situation?

Suggested answers:

- You got it wrong with your stereotyping which is likely to throw you.
- There may be problems with clinical responsibility for her prescription. Why has the supply route changed: was it due to budgetary constraints? Can you prescribe it?
- The patient could become 'piggy in the middle' while you try and resolve the situation with the consultant/manager.
- The conflict is not with the patient in this case but with the hospital.

CASE FOUR

You make a note to yourself to discuss the prescribing situation with your local hospital and settle down to the rest of your surgery. You are still running late when your receptionist calls you to tell you that a Mr Young is at the desk and he is very upset. He is demanding to see you now. He had an appointment at 10.00 and it is now 10.45.

Think about the sources of conflict in this situation.

Suggested answers:

- You have an angry patient on your hands whatever the cause. The situation has to be defused before it escalates.
- Forming any kind of relationship will be a problem: how will you handle him? How will you handle the other patients waiting to see you?
- Fear for self and staff.

> You decide to see him. He comes into your room and before sitting down tells you that he is really angry at the practice and being kept waiting this morning was the last straw.

How do you try and defuse this situation?

Suggested answers:

- Reassure without being too apologetic.
- Use your body language to communicate confidence and a desire to help.
- Allow the patient time to express his concerns – if he calms down you can go on to explore the issues, if not perhaps you can adjourn to later in the day.

> Mr Young calms down and apologises for being so upset. Yesterday morning his son (15) was seen with a painful testicle. The doctor who saw him, your senior partner, told him to take some paracetamol and it would settle down. Last night the duty doctor was called out who admitted him to hospital with a twisted testicle. At operation it was found that it was to late to save the testicle. The surgeon said, 'If he had only come in earlier.'

Think about the conflicts this situation could raise.

Suggested answers:

- Conflict with senior partner.
- Internal conflict – loyalty to patient or partner.
- What action should be taken?
- What do you say to the patient?

CASE FIVE

> Your last patient this morning is a colleague. Dr Williams is a part-
> ner at another practice in town. He is 45, married with two children.
> You know him quite well and play squash with him.

*Think about the possible conflicts that can arise when dealing with a
colleague.*

Suggested answers:

- Relationship – too close to be objective.
- Establishing a working relationship.
- Expectations – does he want you to be a GP or a route for referral?
- Conflict between Dr William's right to confidentiality and his
  patients' safety.

> Dr Williams tells you that he is tired all the time and is suffering
> from insomnia. He keeps getting awful headaches which don't
> respond well to painkillers. He tells you he is scared that he may
> have a brain tumour.

What issues does this raise?

Suggested answers:

- Managing a sick doctor – compliance.
- Patient expectations – differing diagnosis.
- Patient safety – he needs time away from work.
- He may face conflict within his practice if he goes off sick – this
  will compound the problem.

> Later that day your practice manager takes you aside and tells you
> that Dr Williams's practice manager has mentioned to her that he
> has been increasingly late for his surgeries and that two patients had
> said that he smelt of whisky when he visited them.

What issues arise now?

Suggested answers:

- Dr Williams has a problem.

- Relationship – can you/should you address these issues in the next consultation?
- Appropriate referral when expectations are different.
- Patient safety – whose responsibility?

CASE SIX

That afternoon you have a practice meeting; you are in the chair this year. The meeting involves all the doctors and the two practice nurses. Dr Jamison was late again and one of the nurses, Mrs Grant, said that she was far too busy to attend. Your practice manager tells you that the agenda is not ready because she has had no one to type it today.

What signs or symptoms of conflict can you elicit from this scenario?

Suggested answers:

- 'Dr Jamison is late again' – this implies that this is a regular occurrence which may be a symptom of his personality. However he could also be unhappy with his life in the practice and be demonstrating his discontent by being late. He could be a victim of burnout. Additionally, his lateness has an effect upon you and the rest of the team – the constant irritation of his lateness may cause conflict to arise
- 'Mrs Grant was too busy to attend' – this could be genuine but could also be her cry for help. There could be friction between the two nurses; they may not have been consulted regarding the timing of the meeting or the content of the agenda. This issue is probably worth exploring.
- '... she had no-one to type it today' – is this an unusual event? This is an important meeting: What has happened to office priorities? Could it mean some upset in the office? Is someone off sick or is someone being unhelpful? Whatever the case there is something wrong and the situation needs investigating. The meeting will already have been disturbed by the lack of agenda and irritation is in the air.

One of the items on your agenda is clinical audit. This generally produces a lively discussion. Dr Jamison gets quite angry and while thumping the table reiterates his reluctance to do any audit at all because he feels it to be time-consuming and a waste of time. Mrs Reid, your other practice nurse, complains that all she seems to do is collect data: no one tells her what happens to it or what it means.

What do you think is taking place now?

Suggested answers:

- Audit is obviously a controversial topic in your practice and a number of your team are not on board. Dr Jamison is obviously in conflict with the rest of the team on this issue and his problems need addressing if not in the meeting at a later date. I would be suspicious of a stress-related problem given his lateness and anger.
- Mrs Reid has been left out of the loop and is rightly annoyed. This is an opportunity for constructive conflict and the meeting could go on to discuss the nurse's role in audit activities. Because she has had the courage to raise her concerns at the meeting you have the opportunity to move on and to resolve the situation while building a positive atmosphere for the future.

The next item on the agenda is a discussion about continuing education. The senior partner tells the meeting that lunch-time meetings and dinners paid for by drug reps are all he requires. Dr Webster, the newest partner, tries to explain that this type of education does not necessarily address his needs and that she would like the local GP Tutor to visit and to help the practice draw up some learning objectives.

What kind of issues does this raise?

Suggested answers:

- Continuing education is another very threatening topic for a number of GPs. The concept has changed over the years and the thought of needs-based education may threaten an individual's self image and 'face'. The senior partner may feel very threatened by the concept and may react aggressively to any suggestion that the GP tutor visit. The new 'youngster' who is fired with enthusiasm may not understand all the underlying issues and will probably not see the suggestion as anything but commonsense.
- There is also a power/authority issue here. Dr Webster is new and junior with relatively little power within the practice whereas the senior partner has been the authority and power figure for many years. Challenging him may prove very difficult and the issues may be swept under the carpet. The junior partner may then be left to fester until she develops her own case of burnout.

> The meeting discusses the issue fairly calmly but there are obviously a number of unaddressed points lurking beneath the surface. No decision is reached and it is decided that Dr Webster will find out more about the process for next time. The date for the next meeting is decided and just as everybody leaves the room the senior partner tells you that he won't be able to attend the next meeting as he has another commitment.

How are you going to handle the problem?

Suggested answers:

There are two possibilities; either this is a real conflict of dates or the senior partner is unable to face further discussion of the issue and is choosing to opt out. Whatever the next meeting decides he may refuse to participate and leave the rest of the team to go it alone. This is an opportunity to address his fears and to try and regain his confidence. If he is feeling threatened he is likely to be angry and negative about the issue and the person that suggested it. He and the junior partner have different perceptions about continuing education and it will take some work on your part to bring them closer together. You may wish to duck the issue if the senior partner only has a year or two until his retirement or you may wish to allow him to opt out and to undertake his continuing education away from the practice. Either is likely to be rather divisive and is certainly not conducive to good team relationships. Ideally you should look for a way to establish common goals between the two partners. It is likely that they both see continuing education as a necessity, they just have different approaches to the issue. Once common goals have been established you could then work together with them to evolve a way forward.

CASE SEVEN

> Thank goodness that meeting is over! You just have time for a couple of visits before evening surgery. Your first visit request is from the wife of a schizophrenic whom you know well. She says that he has started hearing things again and is reluctant to take his medication.

What problems do you foresee with this visit? What might you do to minimise any risk involved?

Suggested answers:

This is a potentially risky situation. Although you know this patient well his illness makes him potentially violent particularly if he has not been taking his medication again. Why has his wife called during the afternoon – has he threatened her or someone else? Best case – he may be perfectly amenable and may only need his medication topped up. Worst case – if he is violent you may have to take action under the Mental Health Act and you may need the police to assist you.

To minimise risk:

- Tell the practice where you are going and how long you antici-pate being out of contact.
- Take a mobile telephone with you.
- Put your screech alarm in your pocket.
- Have all the telephone numbers you may need to hand.
- Be careful not to let yourself be trapped when you are in the house.

> You get to the flat and find that Mrs Aitken is rather distressed. Her husband thinks that she is poisoning him and he is refusing to take any medication. He refuses to talk to her and is sitting watching the television.

How might you handle the situation – what strategies could you use to minimise the chance of conflict or aggression?

Suggested answers:

Mr Aitken is a member of a subgroup which is more likely to resort to aggression. Your first aim must be self-preservation and you must keep an exit open should he become aggressive or violent. You should not put yourself at a disadvantage. Don't sit down on a soft sofa, either stand or use a hard-backed chair. Use your body lan-guage to defuse the situation. Keep a reasonable distance between you and the patient, keep your hands open and relaxed. Do not frown and keep your face as relaxed as possible. Speak in a clear low voice – do not allow yourself to get involved in a shouting match.

> Your strategies seem to have worked because he agrees to take his medication tonight and to come and see the CPN (community psy-chiatric nurse) in the practice tomorrow. You make a note to brief the team about this appointment.

What issues might you want to raise with the rest of the practice team prior to Mr Aitken's visit?

Suggested answers:

This is a potentially aggressive patient who is visiting the practice. The staff should be aware of that and should activate the protocol for dealing with such patients. He should be dealt with promptly and whenever possible not kept waiting. If necessary he should be moved up waiting lists to prevent problems arising. He should be allowed to sit in an empty consulting room rather than the main waiting area if it is very noisy or busy. The staff should be aware he is in the building and when he is with whoever is seeing him. It is better to plan for the worst case in the hope that the visit will be uneventful.

This may also be a good time to review practice procedures and where necessary update them.

CASE EIGHT

> Your last visit of the day is to Carol Morgan. She is terminally ill with ovarian cancer which has spread widely. Hospital treatment has failed to help and she has been discharged home. You know Carol and her husband well. David has always denied that the disease might kill her while Carol seems to accept the situation with resignation; she just doesn't want to suffer any pain.

What conflicts could arise from this visit?

Suggested answers:

- You may become the target of David's anger as he acknowledges the failure of treatment and Carol's imminent death.
- David may express anger at you and at the hospital for failing to cure Carol.
- How are you going to prevent that happening – counselling David about the situation, try to get him to talk to Carol?
- The management of Carol's pain may cause her not to function so well – David may become angry about this.
- When does controlling pain become more important than preserving life?

> During your visit Carol asks you to make sure that she doesn't suffer. When it all becomes too much she would like you just to 'give her a large injection and finish it off'

How do you avoid conflict with Carol when faced with this request?

Suggested answers:

- Carol has an inaccurate understanding of your abilities.
- Euthanasia is not legal in this country and you need to explain that to Carol very gently.
- Reassure her that you will do your very best to maintain her quality of life right up to the end and that you will try to see that it never 'gets too much'.

Carol dies later that week. David is very angry about her treatment and feels it was the medical profession's fault that she died. He is due to visit the surgery to collect the death certificate.

What strategies can the practice use to minimise the trauma of this visit?

Suggested answers:

- Brief the staff that he is due to visit.
- Make sure that the certificate is readily available and that David will not have to wait.
- If a delay occurs David should be asked to wait in an unoccupied surgery rather than in a noisy waiting room.
- Offer your condolences if appropriate.
- Make sure that all hospital appointments, etc. are notified so that he receives no inappropriate letters.

12. Summary and conclusions

In this chapter we would like to draw together some of the threads of discussion that permeate this book. Conflict is a part of our lives. We see it in the debating chambers of the House of Commons, we see it on the streets of Northern Ireland and we see it in the practices in which we work. There is no aspect of our lives that is free from conflict so we have to learn to deal with it and, wherever possible, deal with it constructively. This book has looked at where we may meet conflict within our work places and also more widely within the context of the National Health Service. Conflict in our practices may not always be avoidable but at the very least we hope that we have given you some strategies with which to attempt to resolve it, or at worst ameliorate its effects.

A PROBLEM

The first step we all have to take in dealing with any problem is to recognise the situation early. There are long lists of symptoms in the book but perhaps the most important aid to recognition is awareness. That is one of the most important lessons you can take from this book. We all dislike conflict and the automatic reaction is to ignore it or to walk away from it. If we continue to do this the problem will almost inevitably escalate and an even worse situation will be left for someone else to manage. Hopefully, with your increased awareness you will be able to identify a potential situation early enough for it to be dealt with.

Having recognised that a problem exists who deals with it? Is it you? The management structure of your workplace will often determine who deals with the problem issues simply because of their position within the hierarchy. However this is not always the case and the responsible manager/partner may be difficult to identify or may lack the authority to take any action. Additionally, they may not be aware that they are the responsible party and if they do not know, how can the rest of the team have any faith in any decision or outcome that they may reach? The responsible manager must not only have the power vested in them to sort out the problem but they must also have the authority to make decisions that the partners and other staff will support. Furthermore, they must have sufficient influence within the workplace to make sure that their team respects and upholds their decisions. Failure to achieve any one of these may result in yet another conflict arising from the attempt to solve the one that has caused the initial problem.

Once you have identified the appropriate manager/partner and given him or her the appropriate delegated authority you need to check that they have the appropriate skills to handle the situation. They must have good communication skills. They must be able to relate to an angry patient and to be understanding with a member of staff who feels aggrieved. They must be able to listen and to hear what all parties are saying. They must also be aware that each combatant has their own view of the problem and that they may be approaching the issue from opposite directions. However much a viewpoint may annoy or irritate, the arbiter must remain non-judgmental and must be seen to be neutral prior to any decision being reached or any action being taken. In essence the person dealing with the problem must be able to recognise their own prejudices (racism, sexism, etc.) and accommodate them.

Having identified the responsible manager he or she may need time to develop the skills to undertake the necessary interviews and counselling. While many doctors have good communication skills and function well within the familiar environment of their surgeries, they often do not function well when trying to arbitrate between two conflicting members of staff. They do not tend to be good judges, usually because it involves taking sides and hurting someone's feelings. Doctors are frequently nice people – it fits with the image of the role! So are managers, but their role image does allow them to deal out unpalatable judgements sometimes. With the appropriate training and support managers are often better able to cope with problem scenarios than are partners.

In dealing with patients, managers often have the advantage. The doctor is often seen as the cause of the patient's problem and as this puts him or her in a negative role acting as arbiter may prove very difficult. The manager is seen as slightly further away from the issue and as a layperson of equal standing to the patient he or she is an appropriate person to deal with the conflict.

Support is important. Conflict tends to cause very negative feelings, ones which we tend to withdraw from or deny. An angry patient or member of staff can be very threatening and if we cannot run from the situation we tend to want to fight back. The managers of problem situations like this, be they practice managers or partners, are definitely moved out of their comfort zones. The situation can cause hurt and anger within those managing it and their stress levels can be very high. Just like the victim of an aggressor, they need debriefing and time to come to terms with their plight.

Stress is very topical and very important. Stress helps us function and indeed it is only with a level of stress that we will function at our best. However, too much stress and we head down the slippery slope. We function less well and become subject to increasing numbers of stress-related illnesses. Practices today should be thinking about stress management at all levels. One man's meat may be another man's poison but the consequences of overload are the same. Management within any practice should include some awareness of the effects of stress and some plans to alleviate its effects at all levels from the cleaner to the senior partner. The senior partner is often the one who catches all the difficult problems but is rarely the one who gets the chance to scream, 'What about me?'

Each staff conflict, every angry patient and every complaint offers an opportunity for learning. These events usually raise powerful emotions and thus are really strong learning tools if used appropriately. If ignored they are strong demotivators and very disruptive. Conflict scenarios cause us to question many of the things we do routinely but we tend to do it in a haphazard fashion and someone always gets blamed for something along the way. Reflection upon any event like this allows us to draw from it the learning messages but few of us find it easy to act in isolation. Critical-event analysis can help draw the team together to reflect and plan.

It is often useful to use a critical event within a practice as an opportunity to reflect upon procedures, training, skills and attitudes. Critical-event analysis can offer a non-threatening framework on which the practice is able hang the events of the crisis and step back to evaluate them. This method allows the practice to study the events for areas which could be approached better or differently and to look for areas where further training might be necessary. Because the session has the potential to be a safe environment it may allow the participants to express deeply held beliefs or attitudes that may be in conflict with their role within the practice. Such situations must be handled carefully and tactfully to avoid another conflict arising. The critical-event analysis allows the practice the opportunity to use the conflict as a base for learning and for moving forward away from the unpleasantness that has overshadowed them.

> Practically, critical-event analysis involves all the involved parties sitting down with the details of the situation and reviewing them and the procedures surrounding them. There is no element of blame to this meeting, it is for purely educational purposes and for the benefit of the practice. It is important that that rule is firmly upheld otherwise input from those who fear repercussions will be distinctly lacking. The leader of the meeting should be responsible for seeing that any actions that seem necessary are investigated and brought to a subsequent meeting when decisions can be made.

One of the consequences of conflict is change. This can be negative or positive; it can range widely, from a practice split to a new set of procedures for filing notes, but it will happen. Change can be highly motivating, but may also be very threatening; unless handled well it can stir up all sorts of issues. It may even result in conflict! Generally, people tend to be suspicious of change and perceive it as devaluing the status quo. That is not necessarily the case: change can be seen as development, as moving towards higher goals albeit a step at a time. Given the threat, however, we, the current managers, must be aware of the issues and must be trained appropriately to handle them. We must also offer our trainees, be they trainee managers or GP registrars, the opportunity to develop the awareness and appropriate skills to deal with these problems when they reach positions of authority.

TO CONCLUDE

Conflict is also a motivator for growth and for change. Our own self-interest requires that we learn to deal with conflict because although we need it to grow and to evolve, we are scared of it and the challenge it brings.

Conflict is not all negative. You may have been involved in a debate or argument which has got particularly heated – often the result of such a situation is to stimulate thought and the critical analysis of a particular viewpoint. New ideas and concepts can be generated, thoughts and ideas can be clarified, any errors or mistakes can be picked up and rectified. However, most of us need a fairly safe environment to expose our feelings, both positive and negative; if our workplace encourages an atmosphere of mutual trust and openness these feelings may be expressed with beneficial consequences.

Our aim in writing this book was to create one port of call to which you could turn when faced with a conflict situation. Although written in the context of general practice much of the information it offers applies to other situations you may encounter. We hope we have offered you some ideas and strategies that will allow you to use conflict positively as a tool with which to help you expand and grow. The book does not cover every issue on the subject but provides a little food for the plant; a little help upon your way.

Index